T0324067

Sarcopenia

Guest Editor

YVES ROLLAND, MD, PhD

CLINICS IN GERIATRIC MEDICINE

www.geriatric.theclinics.com

August 2011 • Volume 27 • Number 3

SAUNDERS an imprint of ELSEVIER, Inc.

W.B. SAUNDERS COMPANY
A Division of Elsevier Inc.

1600 John F. Kennedy Blvd., Suite 1800. Philadelphia, Pennsylvania 19103-2899

http://www.theclinics.com

CLINICS IN GERIATRIC MEDICINE Volume 27, Number 3
August 2011 ISSN 0749–0690, ISBN-13: 978-1-4557-0454-5

Editor: Yonah Korngold
Developmental Editor: Donald E. Mumford

Clinics in Geriatric Medicine (ISSN 0749-0690) is published quarterly by Elsevier Inc., 360 Park Avenue South, New York, NY 10010-1710. Months of issue are February, May, August, and November. Business and Editorial Offices: 1600 John F. Kennedy Blvd., Suite 1800, Philadelphia, PA 191023-2899. Periodicals postage paid at New York, NY, and additional mailing offices. Subscription prices is $241.00 per year (US individuals), $427.00 per year (US institutions), $123.00 per year (US student/resident), $314.00 per year (Canadian individuals), $532.00 per year (Canadian institutions), $333.00 per year (foreign individuals) and $532.00 per year (foreign institutions). Foreign air speed delivery is included in all *Clinics* subscription prices. All prices are subject to change without notice. POSTMASTER: Send address changes to *Clinics in Geriatric Medicine*, Elsevier Health Sciences Division, Subscription Customer Service, 3251 Riverport Lane, Maryland Heights, MO 63043. Telephone: 1-800-654-2452 (U.S. and Canada); 314-447-8871 (outside U.S. and Canada). Fax: 314-447-8029. E-mail: journalscustomerservice-usa@elsevier.com (for print support) or journalsonlinesupport-usa@elsevier.com (for online support).

Reprints. For copies of 100 or more, of articles in this publication, please contact the Commercial Reprints Department, Elsevier Inc., 360 Park Avenue South, New York, New York 10010-1710. Tel.: (212) 633-3812; Fax: (212) 462-1935, email: reprints@elsevier.com.

Clinics in Geriatric Medicine is covered in *MEDLINE/PubMed (Index Medicus), EMBASE/Excerpta Medica, Current Contents/Clinical Medicine (CC/CM), and the Cumulative Index to Nursing & Allied Health Literature.*

Printed in the United States of America.

Contributors

GUEST EDITOR

YVES ROLLAND, MD, PhD
Professor of Geriatrics, INSERM U1027, University of Toulouse III, Toulouse; Gérontopôle de Toulouse, Department of Medicine, Toulouse University Hospital, Toulouse, France

AUTHORS

JUERGEN M. BAUER, MD
Associate Professor, Direktor der Klinik für Geriatrie, Leiter des Geriatrischen Zentrums Oldenburg (GZO), Oldenburg, Germany

RICHARD N. BAUMGARTNER, PhD
Professor and Chair, Department of Epidemiology and Population Health, University of Louisville, Louisville, Kentucky

YVES BOIRIE, MD, PhD
Professor of Nutrition, Clinical Nutrition Department, University Hospital of Clermont-Ferrand; Human Nutrition Unit, Clermont-Ferrand, France

NOËL CANO, MD, PhD
INRA; Université Clermont 1, UFR de Médecine; Service de Nutrition Clinique, CHU Clermont-Ferrand, Hôpital Gabriel Montpied, Clermont-Ferrand, France

GILLES CARNAC, PhD
Scientific Researcher, French National Institute for Health and Medical Research (INSERM), Montpellier, France

TOMMY E. CEDERHOLM, MD, PhD
Professor of Clinical Nutrition and Senior Consultant, Clinical Nutrition and Metabolism, Department of Public Health and Caring Sciences, Uppsala University; Department of Geriatrics, University Hospital, Uppsala, Sweden

WM. CAMERON CHUMLEA, MD, PhD
Lifespan Health Research Center, Department of Community Health, Boonshoft School of Medicine, Wright State University, Dayton, Ohio

CHARLOTTE DUPUY, MSPT
Gérontopôle de Toulouse, Department of Geriatric Medicine, Toulouse University Hospital; INSERM, University Toulouse-III, Toulouse, France

SOPHIE GILLETTE-GUYONET, PhD
Gérontopôle de Toulouse, Department of Geriatric Medicine, Toulouse University Hospital, Toulouse; INSERM U1027, University of Toulouse III, Toulouse, France

CHRISTELLE GUILLET, PhD
INRA; Université Clermont 1, UFR de Médecine, Clermont-Ferrand, France

MATHIEU HOULES, MD
Gérontopôle de Toulouse, Department of Geriatric Medicine, Toulouse University Hospital, Toulouse, France

IAN JANSSEN, PhD
Associate Professor and CRC Chair in Physical Activity and Obesity, School of Kinesiology and Health Studies, Department of Community Health and Epidemiology, Queen's University, Kingston, Ontario, Canada

DALILA LAOUDJ-CHENIVESSE, PhD
Scientific Researcher, French National Institute for Health and Medical Research (INSERM); Scientific Researcher, Medical University of Montpellier, Montpellier, France

JACQUES MERCIER, MD, PhD
Professor of Medicine, Physiologist, French National Institute for Health and Medical Research (INSERM); Medical University of Montpellier; University Hospital of Montpellier, Montpellier, France

JOHN E. MORLEY, MD, PhD
Professor of Geriatric Medicine, Geriatric Research, Education and Clinical Center, St Louis Veterans Affairs Medical Center; Division of Geriatrics, St Louis University School of Medicine, St Louis, Missouri

GRAZIANO ONDER, MD, PhD
Professor of Geriatric Medicine, Department of Gerontology and Geriatrics, Catholic University of Sacred Heart, Rome, Italy

FABIEN PILLARD, MD, PhD
Doctor of Medicine, Respiratory Exploration Department and Sports Medicine Department, University Hospital of Toulouse; Physiologist, Physiology Department, Medical University of Toulouse III; French National Institute for Health and Medical Research (INSERM), Obesity Research Unit, Toulouse, France

JACQUES RAMI, PhD
Physiologist, Scientific Researcher, Respiratory Exploration Department and Sports Medicine Department, University Hospital of Toulouse; Physiology Department, Medical University of Toulouse III; French National Institute for Health and Medical Research (INSERM), Obesity Research Unit, Toulouse, France

DANIEL RIVIÈRE, MD, PhD
Professor of Medicine, Physiologist, Respiratory Exploration Department and Sports Medicine Department, University Hospital of Toulouse; Physiology Department, Medical University of Toulouse III; French National Institute for Health and Medical Research (INSERM), Obesity Research Unit, Toulouse, France

YVES ROLLAND, MD, PhD
Professor of Geriatrics, INSERM U1027, University of Toulouse III, Toulouse; Gérontopôle de Toulouse, Department of Medicine, Toulouse University Hospital, Toulouse, France

IRWIN H. ROSENBERG, MD
Jean Mayer University Professor, Tufts University, Boston, Massachusetts

JÉROME SALLES, PhD
INRA, Université Clermont 1, UFR de Médecine, Clermont-Ferrand, France

LAURA A. SCHAAP, PhD
EMGO+ Institute and Department of Epidemiology and Biostatistics, VU University Medical Center, Amsterdam, The Netherlands

STEPHANE M. SCHNEIDER, MD, PhD
Professor of Nutrition, Nutritional Support Unit, Archet University Hospital, University of Nice Sophia-Antipolis, Nice, France

CORNEL C. SIEBER, MD
Professor of Medicine, Chair Internal Medicine-Geriatrics, Director, Institute for Biomedicine of Aging, Friedrich-Alexander-Universität Erlangen-Nürnberg, Nürnberg, Germany

GABOR ABELLAN VAN KAN, MD
Professor of Geriatric Medicine, INSERM U1027, University of Toulouse III, Toulouse; Gérontopôle de Toulouse, Department of Geriatric Medicine, Toulouse University Hospital, Toulouse, France

BRUNO VELLAS, MD, PhD
Professor of Geriatric Medicine, INSERM U1027, University of Toulouse III, Toulouse; Gérontopôle de Toulouse, Department of Geriatric Medicine, Toulouse University Hospital, Toulouse, France

MARJOLEIN VISSER, PhD
Department of Health Sciences, Faculty of Earth and Life Sciences, VU University Amsterdam; EMGO+ Institute and Department of Epidemiology and Biostatistics, VU University Medical Center, Amsterdam, The Netherlands

STÉPHANE WALRAND, PhD
INRA; Université Clermont 1, UFR de Médecine, Clermont-Ferrand, France

DEBRA L. WATERS, PhD
Senior Lecturer, Department of Preventive and Social Medicine, Dunedin School of Medicine, University of Otago, Dunedin, New Zealand

Contents

To a considerable extent, the advent of the term sarcopenia has contributed to the focus on this important condition and its effects on the quality of life and care of older persons. It is hoped that the advances in our understanding of the etiology and treatment of sarcopenia will further contribute to placing this diagnosis and treatment at a higher priority in the management of older persons and prevention of disability.

The definition of sarcopenia has been thoroughly discussed by scientific stakeholders and industry representatives to increase the clinical applicability of the concept. The pooled consensus from 3 of 5 recent and parallel processes, of which 2 are pending, is that sarcopenia is mainly, but not only, an age-related condition defined by the combined presence of reduced muscle mass and muscle function. Contributing factors to sarcopenia are senescence, chronic disease, physical inactivity, and poor food intake. Cachexia may be considered as one etiologic pathway of an accelerated sarcopenia. The adjusted and extended definitions of sarcopenia promote the clinical use of the concept.

The term sarcopenia was coined in 1989 and refers to the age-related loss in skeletal muscle mass. Operational definitions of sarcopenia have been used in research studies to identify older persons with healthy muscle mass values (normal) and older adults with unacceptably low muscle mass values (sarcopenic). Despite the enormous research on sarcopenia that has been completed in the past 20 years, sarcopenia currently receives little attention in the clinical setting. To address this issue, the European Working Group on Sarcopenia in Older People recently developed a consensus definition of sarcopenia. The availability of a consensus definition may assist with the integration of sarcopenia into mainstream geriatric assessment.

The etiology of sarcopenia is multifactorial but still poorly understood, and the sequelae of this phenomenon represent a major public health issue.

Age-related loss of muscle mass can be counteracted by adequate metabolic interventions including nutritional intake and exercise training. Other strategies including changes in daily protein pattern, the speed of protein digestion, or specific amino acid supplementation may be beneficial to improve short-term muscle anabolic response in elderly people. A multimodal approach combining nutrition, exercise, hormones, and specific anabolic drugs may be an innovative treatment for limiting the development of sarcopenia with aging.

This article describes the relationship of sarcopenia and dynapenia with three important outcomes in aging research: functional status, falls, and mortality. The data from epidemiologic studies conducted in large samples of older men and women suggest that muscle functioning, as indicated by muscle strength or muscle power, has a strong impact on functional status, falls, and mortality. Furthermore, there is evidence that the relationship between poor muscle strength and these three different outcomes is not influenced by muscle size. For the prevention of functional decline, falls, and early mortality in older men and women a major focus on maintaining or increasing muscle strength instead of muscle size seems warranted.

Four body composition phenotypes exist in older adults: normal, sarcopenic, obese, and a combination of sarcopenic and obese. There is no consensus, however, on the definitions and classifications of these phenotypes and their etiology and consequences continue to be debated. The lack of standard definitions, particularly for sarcopenia and sarcopenic obesity, creates challenges for determining prevalence across different populations. The etiology of these phenotypes is multifactorial with complex covariate relationships. This review focuses on the current literature addressing the classification, prevalence, etiology, and correlates of sarcopenia, obesity, and the combination of sarcopenia and obesity, referred to as sarcopenic obesity.

Sarcopenia is a complex multifactorial condition that can by treated with multimodal approaches. No pharmacologic agent to prevent or treat sarcopenia has been as efficacious as exercise (mainly resistance training) in combination with nutritional intervention (adequate protein and energy intake). However, performing resistance training sessions and following nutritional advice can be challenging, especially for frail, sarcopenic, elderly patients, and results remain only partial. Therefore, new pharmacologic agents may substantially reduce the functional decline in older people. This article reviews the new pharmacologic agents currently being assessed for treating sarcopenia.

Fabien Pillard, Dalila Laoudj-Chenivesse, Gilles Carnac, Jacques Mercier, Jacques Rami, Daniel Rivière, and Yves Rolland

Physical activity can be a valuable countermeasure to sarcopenia in its treatment and prevention. In considering physical training strategies for sarcopenic subjects, it is critical to consider personal and environmental obstacles to access opportunities for physical activity for any patient with chronic disease. This article presents an overview of current knowledge of the effects of physical training on muscle function and the physical activity recommended for sarcopenic patients. So that this countermeasure strategy can be applied in practice, the authors propose a standardized protocol for prescribing physical activity in chronic diseases such as sarcopenia.

Gabor Abellan van Kan, WM. Cameron Chumlea, Sophie Gillette-Guyonet, Mathieu Houles, Charlotte Dupuy, Yves Rolland, and Bruno Vellas

Phase 3 trials estimate the effectiveness of an intervention to prevent, delay the onset of, or treat sarcopenia. Participants should have sarcopenia or present a sarcopenia risk profile. Control group should be characterized by the best standard of clinical care. This article further develops issues on sarcopenia definition, target population, primary and secondary end points, duration of the trials, muscle mass assessment, strength and physical performance assessment, and control of possible confounders. The challenges to conduct phase 3 trials in the elderly should not offset the opportunities for the development of new strategies to counteract sarcopenia and prevent late-life disability.

THE CLINICS ARE NOW AVAILABLE ONLINE!

Access your subscription at:
www.theclinics.com

Preface

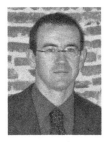

Yves Rolland, MD, PhD
Guest Editor

Sarcopenia, a progressive reduction in skeletal muscle mass, strength, and quality, is often observed with aging. This condition is one of the main factors that contribute to frailty in older adults. During the past 10 years, sarcopenia has received growing attention by both clinicians and researchers. Indeed, it results in poor physical performances, decreased endurance and resistance capacity, and increased risk of falls and fractures that all contribute to the loss of independence. Sarcopenia also has a deleterious effect on metabolism related to the changes in body composition. Compared to other changes of body composition observed during aging, such as obesity or osteoporosis, sarcopenia was only recently defined but has now emerged as a major public health problem.

Today, a lot more is known about the causes, consequences, and the current and potential future treatment of sarcopenia. In this special issue of the *Clinics in Geriatric Medicine*, authors provide insight into the mechanism by which sarcopenia impairs physical function and the quality of life in older people. These articles are encouraging and suggest that there is some promise for efficacy in new approaches. Recent scientific findings also provide the framework for the use of new nutritional approaches (such as essential amino acid supplementation) and physical exercise in order to improve muscular tissue.

The functional decline observed in the elderly population should no longer be judged with fatalism. The field of study on sarcopenia is a huge opportunity to organize clinical interventions to benefit the frail older person. We hope that this special issue on sarcopenia will help clinicians and researchers better understand this new area of investigation and improve their ability to preserve independence in the elderly population.

Yves Rolland, MD, PhD
Service de Médecine Interne et de Gérontologie Clinique
INSERM 1027 Pavillon Junod, 170 avenue de Casselardit
Hôpital La Grave-Casselardit
31300 Toulouse, France

E-mail address:
rolland.y@chu-toulouse.fr

Clin Geriatr Med 27 (2011) xi
doi:10.1016/j.cger.2011.04.002   geriatric.theclinics.com
0749-0690/11/$ – see front matter © 2011 Elsevier Inc. All rights reserved.

Sarcopenia: Origins and Clinical Relevance

Irwin H. Rosenberg, MD

• Sarcopenia • Aging • Muscle • Strength

The term sarcopenia is barely more than 20 years old. Sarcopenia has been most recently defined by a group of scientists composing an international working group as "the age-associated loss of skeletal muscle mass and function,"[1] which adopted a definition put forward earlier by the author and his colleagues stating that sarcopenia refers specifically to "involuntary loss of skeletal muscle mass and consequently of strength."[2] Those working in the field of geriatrics and in the care of the elderly may be curious about the origin of this term and may even wonder about the need for a current consensus definition some 20 years after the term was first applied to this important condition in aging in remarks at a meeting about the epidemiology of aging in Albuquerque, New Mexico in 1989.[3] However, the phenomenon of loss of muscle strength, and even muscle mass, with aging was observed years earlier in 1931 when Critchley[4] noted that muscle loss occurs with aging, and the process of loss of certain fiber types in human skeletal muscle over time was observed in studies of muscle biopsies, even after the first few decades of life.[5] A dramatic age-associated decline in world weight-lifting records between 30 and 60 years of age that was attributable to loss of muscle strength and power, beginning as early as 35 years of age, was also observed.[6] Truly, the history of sarcopenia is as old as the aging of man, even if the term sarcopenia is but 20 years old.

The meeting in Albuquerque, at which the author first used the term sarcopenia in the summary comments,[3] was one effort to collect information about the population distribution of conditions associated with aging. Many of these functional changes with age were discussed by Nathan Shock[7] based on his cross-sectional studies in Baltimore of declines in many different functions over the age span, including sensory, cardiovascular, respiratory, and renal function. The prevalence of some of these declines in older populations was described at the Albuquerque meeting, along with a strong emphasis on the loss of bone mineral mass with age, as a basis for the increasingly recognized problem of osteoporosis. Colleagues at the USDA Human

Statement acknowledging funding support: N/A.
Conflict of interest and financial disclosure: The author has nothing to disclose.
Tufts University, 150 Harrison Avenue, Jaharis Building, Boston, MA 02111, USA
E-mail address: Irwin.rosenberg@tufts.edu

Clin Geriatr Med 27 (2011) 337–339
doi:10.1016/j.cger.2011.03.003   geriatric.theclinics.com
0749-0690/11/$ – see front matter © 2011 Elsevier Inc. All rights reserved.

Nutrition Research Center on Aging at Tufts University, especially William Evans, were interested in changes in body composition over time and others reflected on the relationship between a change in body weight and possibly lean mass affecting basal metabolic weight, as a basis for decline in appetite with age. There was also emerging evidence that a decline in muscle mass over time indicated by declining urinary creatinine was associated with declining physical activity and strength, as well as decline in basal metabolic rate. There was already evidence that some of the frailty and loss of mobility and balance concomitant with loss of muscle strength with aging was an increasingly recognized cause for admission to the hospital and nursing home care and general loss of independence. The author's comments at that meeting were in the form of a question: why were we spending so much of our concentration on loss of bone mass when there was burgeoning evidence that the loss of muscle mass and strength might be every bit as important as a cause of disability among elders? The author proposed the term sarcopenia to capture the Greek meanings of "sarco" (flesh or muscle) and "penia" (loss). The author proposed somewhat jokingly that it might be necessary for there to be a Greek term for this condition in parallel with osteoporosis or osteopenia in order that it be taken seriously.

The issue of what will be taken seriously by the research community, the practicing community, and by funding sources is more than a trivial matter. As an example, we have seen a burst of interest in research in age-related cognitive decline when use of the term Alzheimer's disease made this important and widespread phenomenon a disease and not just a concomitant of aging. So, we saw a rapid acceptance of the need for more research and concentration on age-related muscle decline when it had the more formal name sarcopenia. It is quite remarkable that within a year of the publication of the leading report, which first used the term sarcopenia, there was a call for research proposals on sarcopenia emanating from the US National Institute of Health (NIH) and particularly the National Institute on Aging. A workshop on sarcopenia at the NIH followed soon after. The first research program dedicated to the study of sarcopenia quickly followed at the Human Nutrition Research Center on Aging, called The Laboratory of Nutrition, Exercise, Physical Activity, and Sarcopenia.

Why is this history important and why is a consensus definition important? One answer may be that the phenomenon of age-related loss of muscle mass and strength has still not been embraced with the deserved priority by the geriatric practice community, even though the broader concept of frailty has been emphasized. Even as the evidence mounts that loss of muscle mass and function may reach levels where mobility and balance are so impaired and falls so prevalent that independence is seriously hampered and institutionalization required, the diagnosis and treatment of sarcopenia is not a standard part of the geriatric care repertoire in the United States, although there appears to be more acceptance in European geriatric circles. This circumstance may be partly caused by the fact that the verbal definition and even the etiologic definition of sarcopenia have not been matched by a consensus on which measurements need to be used in defining and diagnosing sarcopenia in the clinical setting. That process has been greatly added to by the consensus group that met in Rome in 2009,[1] and that may be a major step in the direction of defining sarcopenia as a disease and condition that can be diagnosed and managed.

There is an additional challenge of understanding the cause and the direction of treatment for this condition and the extent to which the loss of function and mass is reversible. These challenges are continuing for both the research and, the clinical community; also needed is the adoption of the current consensus definition. My colleagues and I proposed a schema for considering the causes of sarcopenia that can also serve as a basis for interventions to ameliorate the effects of muscle loss

---

Box 1
Etiologic factors in sarcopenia

- Inactivity
- Increased muscle fat
- Insulin resistance
- Loss of alpha motor neurons
- Decreased dieting intake (of protein?)
- Increased interleukin-6
- Loss of estrogen or androgen
- Decreased growth hormone secretion

Data from Roubenoff R, Heymsfield S, Kehayias J, et al. Standardization of nomenclature of body composition in weight loss. Am J Clin Nutr 1997;66:192–6.

---

and weakness. The list of interacting factors hypothesized or accepted as elements in the etiology of sarcopenia are listed in **Box 1**. This list demands further elucidation and provides more targets for ongoing research.

We know from the pioneering work of Fiatarone[8] and Fielding[1] that resistance exercise, exercise with nutritional supplementation are modalities that can effect and reverse the muscle loss and substantially improve muscle strength and mobility and balance. If we are to further capture the attention of geriatric practitioners and others who care for the elderly, we must continue to advance our knowledge on both the etiology and treatment and the reversal of sarcopenia.

To a considerable extent, the advent of the term sarcopenia has contributed to the focus on this important condition and its effects on the quality of life and care of older persons. It is hoped that the advances in our understanding of the etiology and treatment of sarcopenia will further contribute to placing this diagnosis and treatment at a higher priority in the management of older persons and prevention of disability.

REFERENCES

1. Fielding R, Vellas B, Evans W, et al. Sarcopenia: an undiagnosed condition in older adults. Current consensus definition: prevalence, etiology, and consequences. J Am Med Dir Assoc 2011;12:249–56.
2. Roubenoff R, Heymsfield S, Kehayias J, et al. Standardization of nomenclature of body composition in weight loss. Am J Clin Nutr 1997;66:192–6.
3. Rosenberg IH. Summary comments. Am J Clin Nutr 1989;50(Suppl):1231S–3S.
4. Critchley M. The neurology of old age. Lancet 1931;1:1221–30.
5. Lexell J, Henriksson-Larsen K, Wimbold B, et al. Distribution of different fiber types in human skeletal muscles: effects of the aging studied in whole muscle cross sections. Muscle Nerve 1983;6:588–95.
6. Available at: www.mastersweightlifting.org/records.htm. Accessed March 21, 2011.
7. Shock NW. Age changes in some physiologic processes. Geriatrics 1957;12:40–8.
8. Fiatarone MA, O'Neill EF, Ryan ND, et al. Exercise training and nutritional supplementation for physical frailty in very elderly people. N Engl J Med 1994;330: 1769–75.

Toward a Definition of Sarcopenia

Tommy E. Cederholm, MD, PhD[a,b],*, Juergen M. Bauer, MD[c],
Yves Boirie, MD, PhD[d,e], Stephane M. Schneider, MD, PhD[f],
Cornel C. Sieber, MD[g], Yves Rolland, MD, PhD[h,i,j]

KEYWORDS

• Sarcopenia • Muscle mass • Aging • Cachexia

THE RELEVANCE OF SARCOPENIA IN THE AGING WORLD

The capacity to live independently is crucial for good quality of life at all ages. With increasing age, this competence is threatened by degenerative processes linked to aging per se, superimposed by incident diseases accumulating during the course of life. Apart from disease, cognitive impairment and muscular dysfunction are the grimmest intimidations of an independent lifestyle at older age. Although the devastating

Disclosure: Studies and talks for Nutricia/Danone, Nestlé, Fresenius-Kabi, and Merck-Sharpe-Dome (T.E.C.). Studies for Nutricia/Danone and Nestlé, talks for Nestlé and Abbott, and consulting and syllabus for Abbott (J.M.B.). Studies, talks, and consulting for Danone and studies for Lactalis (Y.B.). Studies and talks for Nutricia/Danone, talks for Nestlé, and consulting and syllabus for Abbott (S.M.S.). Studies, talks, and consulting for Nestlé; studies and talks for Danone; and syllabus for Abbott (C.C.S.). Studies and talks for Lactalis, Lundbeck, MSD, Danone, Lilly, and Cheisi (Y.R.).

[a] Clinical Nutrition and Metabolism, Department of Public Health and Caring Sciences, Uppsala University, Uppsala Science Park, Dag Hammarskjöldsväg 14B, 75185 Uppsala, Sweden
[b] Department of Geriatrics, University Hospital, 75185 Uppsala, Sweden
[c] Klinik fur Geriatrie, Geriatrischen Zentrums Oldenburg (GZO), Rahel-Straus-Strasse 10, 26133 Oldenburg, Germany
[d] Clinical Nutrition Department, University Hospital of Clermont-Ferrand, 58 rue Montalembert, BP 69, 63003 Clermont-Ferrand CEDEX, France
[e] Human Nutrition Unit, 58, rue Montalembert BP 321, 63009 Clermont-Ferrand, France
[f] Nutritional Support Unit, Archet University Hospital, University of Nice Sophia-Antipolis, 261 Route de Grenoble, 06205 Nice, France
[g] Institute for Biomedicine of Aging, Friedrich-Alexander-Universität Erlangen-Nürnberg, Ernst-Nathan-Strasse 1, 90419 Nürnberg, Germany
[h] Inserm U1027; F-31073, Avenue Jules Guesdes, University of Toulouse III, F-31073, France
[i] Avenue Jules Guesdes, University of Toulouse III, Toulouse, France
[j] Gérontopôle de Toulouse, Pavillon Junod, 170 avenue de Casselardit, Toulouse University Hospital, 31300 Toulouse, France
* Corresponding author. Clinical Nutrition and Metabolism, Department of Public Health and Caring Sciences, Uppsala University, Uppsala Science Park, Dag Hammarskjöldsväg 14B, 75185 Uppsala, Sweden.
E-mail address: tommy.cederholm@pubcare.uu.se

Clin Geriatr Med 27 (2011) 341–353
doi:10.1016/j.cger.2011.04.001
0749-0690/11/$ – see front matter
geriatric.theclinics.com

effects of Alzheimer disease and osteoporosis have been focused on during the past decades, the frailty cornerstones of fatigue, weakness, and low physical activity (ie, reduced muscle function) have not gained as much attention. The concept of sarcopenia, that is, Greek for muscle loss, was introduced by concerned physicians in the late 1980s in an attempt to increase awareness of age-related muscle loss and its shattering effects on the freedom of the elderly. Rosenberg[1] wrote in 1989, "There may be no single feature of age-related decline that could so dramatically affect ambulation, mobility, independence and breathing. Why have we not given it more attention? Perhaps it needs a name derived from the Greek. I'll suggest a couple: sarcomalacia or sarcopenia." According to the remarkable ongoing global demographic shift, this suggestion was, is, and will be of utmost significance for the medical community that strives to improve functionality and quality of life for older individuals.

The proportion of the aged population is growing fast. During the twentieth century, median life span increased by 30 years in the Western world.[2] The United Nations has projected that until 2030, the global population aged 60 years and older will grow almost 4 times faster than the total population.[3] Provided that this process continues uninterruptedly, it has been anticipated that more than half of the newborns of today will live to experience their 100th birthday.[2] This extreme shift of demography presents a major challenge to the society. The degenerative features of aging that daunt independent living at old age are governed by genetic, environmental, and lifestyle factors. The environmental and lifestyle factors can be addressed by society and on an individual basis as well. Measures are urgently needed.

EARLY CONCEPTS OF SARCOPENIA

Sarcopenia has become a core concept for understanding the necessary course of action to maintain good function at old age. Muscle accounts for about 40% and 75% of body mass and body cell mass, respectively.[4] In the early years after 1990, sarcopenia was defined as the decline in muscle mass and function seen during aging, "the term actually describes an important change in body composition and function,"[5] or as "the age-related loss in skeletal muscle mass, which results in decreased strength and aerobic capacity and thus functional capacity."[6] The scientific community adopted the concept, and research aiming at the understanding of the relevant pathogenic mechanisms was launched.[6–8]

SENESCENCE AND SARCOPENIA

At this stage, research was focused on the mechanisms triggered by senescence. Longitudinal studies on urinary creatinine excretion in healthy people had indicated a reduced muscle mass of up to 50% between 20 and 80 years of age.[9] After age 50 years, about 1% to 2% of muscle mass is projected to be lost per year.[10] Muscle strength is lost at an even greater pace.[11] Cross-sectional studies indicated that young men have twice as much muscle mass as fat mass, whereas older men's muscle mass-to-fat mass ratio is almost reversed, although maintaining comparable body mass index (BMI) values.[12] Early data suggested that mainly the fast type II fibers decrease in numbers and size during aging.[13–16] This decrease could be induced by increased susceptibility, especially in type II fibers, to apoptosis caused by frequent mutations in mitochondrial DNA and caspase activation.[17] Physical inactivity in later life offers another explanation because a sedentary lifestyle only rarely activates the strong type II fibers, which thus may undergo inactivity-induced atrophy. During aging, there is a progressive denervation process affecting axons of alpha motor neurons.[18] The enlarged motor neuron territories result in deterioration of muscle coordination and decreased strength.[19] Reduced secretion of anabolic hormones,[20] such as testosterone and dehydroepiandrostenedione, as well as growth hormones, such as somatotropin and insulinlike growth factor 1, is controlled genetically.

Systemic inflammation, for example, elevated activity of tumor necrosis factor α and interleukin 1 among many cytokines, leads to muscle protein breakdown. Although disease is the major cause of inflammation in older age, aging itself (inflammaging[21]) is also linked to muscle catabolic chronic low-grade inflammation.[22] The search for the molecular basis of inflammation-triggered muscle atrophy has rendered the discovery of upregulated genes of E3 ubiquitin ligases MuRF1 and Atrogin-1, which are both involved in the activation of the ubiquitin-proteasome system and the muscle fiber actin and myosin proteolyses.[23–25] In contrast to disease-triggered muscle wasting being dominated by protein breakdown, senescence-related muscle atrophy is suggested to be mainly an effect of reduced protein synthesis, especially in response to feeding.[26] The molecular basis of such perturbed signaling pathways involves the action of the mammalian target of rapamycin (mTOR) kinase, which is recognized as a key regulator of cell growth. mTOR is a sensor of nutritional status and may play a role as a potential target of amino acid–induced protein synthesis.[25,27]

Satellite cell dysfunction is an emerging field of improved molecular understanding of the development of sarcopenia.[28] Satellite cells are myogenic stem cells that merge with myocytes and differentiate into new muscle fibers. Myostatin D is a recently described molecule that inhibits the generation of satellite cells.[29] These cells also have the capacity to become adipocytes and thus are involved in the development of myosteatosis,[30] that is, fat infiltration of aging muscles.

Insulin resistance, partly because of inflammaging, contributes to muscle wasting.[31] Obesity and myosteatosis are additional causes of insulin resistance because intra-myocellular lipid accumulation may impair insulin signaling not only for glucose but also for amino acid utilization by skeletal muscle.[32] Although muscle mass decreases during aging, the relative, and sometimes also the absolute, amount of fat mass increases. Thus, weight may be unchanged or even increased, resulting in a condition that has been called sarcopenic obesity.[33] This transition of body composition fuels a vicious cycle of insulin resistance and further loss of muscle mass.

CACHEXIA, WASTING DISORDER, AND SARCOPENIA

During the 1980s and 1990s, a progressive understanding of protein-energy malnutrition (PEM) in various clinical contexts developed. High prevalence in hospitals and especially in nursing homes was reported, and efforts to understand the underlying mechanisms were commenced. It was agreed on that PEM was not a homogenous entity. This understanding initially emanated from the cancer field. Cancer-induced PEM was found to be strongly associated with inflammatory processes.[34,35] Although this scenario was particularly relevant for cancer, it gradually became clear that most disease-related forms of PEM were related to increased cytokine activity,[36–38] which is responsible for anorexia, hypermetabolism, and muscle proteolysis.[39] Moreover, it was observed that PEM with elevated inflammatory activity only weakly responded to nutritional treatment.[40,41]

Because of such understanding, a new terminology was suggested in 1997.[42] Cachexia was introduced as the disease-related loss of body cell mass, not necessarily linked with concurrent weight loss. Weight loss irrespective of the effects on body composition was called wasting disorder, whereas the involuntary, age-associated, non–disease-related, that is, age-specific, muscle loss was called sarcopenia.

The term wasting disorder turned out to be difficult to translate into wordings understandable by those outside the English-speaking medical community. English medical terms are usually not accepted in non–English-speaking countries, whereas Greek or Latin terms are. Also, the general term muscle loss or muscle wasting induced a linguistic predicament because few languages have specific wordings for this condition, which could be adequately interpreted by the medical community. Cachexia is often wrongly used as a proxy for extreme emaciation.

Nevertheless, the suggested terminology of 1997 encouraged research into the deeper understanding of disease-related catabolism and the mechanisms involved in muscle wasting.[43–46] The molecular basis for inflammatory-triggered perturbation of muscle synthesis and breakdown was investigated and better understood.[24,25,47]

SARCOPENIA ON THE EPIDEMIOLOGIC SCENE

After the publication of the definition of sarcopenia in 1997, several population-based, mainly American, cohorts were used to assess the prevalence of sarcopenia. Criteria for sarcopenia were mainly defined in analogy to osteoporosis, that is, a T score of reduced muscle mass. Accordingly, muscle mass below 2 SDs of mean muscle mass in a healthy young reference population was used as the cutoff. The estimation of muscle mass depends on measurement techniques, for example, dual-energy x-ray absorptiometry (DXA) or bioelectrical impedance analysis (BIA), if whole-body or appendicular muscle mass is used and if muscle mass is related to height, body mass, or fat mass. The studies from New Mexico, using appendicular fat-free mass, measured by DXA and divided by height squared, described the prevalence of sarcopenia to be around 10% to 20% for those younger than 80 years and close to 30% for those older than 80 years.[48–50] In the National Health and Nutrition Examination Survey III cohort, the prevalence was suggested to be around 10% among those older than 60 years.[51] The data were derived from measurements of whole-body skeletal muscle mass by BIA[52] and divided by body mass. In addition and in the same cohort, BIA-derived absolute muscle mass was normalized for height squared, and cut points for questionnaire-based evaluation of high physical disability risk were suggested to be 5.75 kg muscle/m^2 or less and 8.5 kg muscle/m^2 or less for women and men, respectively.[53] The data from the Health Aging and Body Composition (ABC) cohorts also indicated that around 20% to 30% of the population between the ages of 70 and 80 years had sarcopenia[54] when appendicular muscle mass was measured by DXA but varied with the technique for normalization. Sarcopenia was more prevalent when BMI was less than 25 kg/m^2. There is no general consensus on how to measure muscle mass, and the assessment of sarcopenia varies with access to body imaging techniques and relevant reference populations.

Population-based cohorts are compiled of mixes of older individuals with widely differing functionality and health status. Information on comorbidities or other potential underlying factors beyond aging per se was not considered in any of these cohort studies. Thus, the given prevalence figures could not be interpreted to relate specifically to age-specific sarcopenia. People with muscle wasting caused by chronic disease, that is, cachexia, and other non–age-specific phenomena, such as sedentarism and insufficient food intake, were most likely abundant in these cohorts.

SARCOPENIA: A GERONTOLOGICAL OR CLINICAL CONCEPT?

When research activities began to approach the clinical arena, with the aim to transfer the acquired knowledge into clinical practice, problems with a mere age-specific definition of sarcopenia became apparent. Such a pure definition is based on the assumption that an affected individual does not suffer from clinical causes that lead to muscle wasting. So far, there are no reliable markers that distinguish true age-specific sarcopenia from other forms of muscle wasting, including cachexia.

Pure age-specific sarcopenia may be regarded as a pronounced manifestation of physiologic aging. Under these circumstances, sarcopenia becomes a research entity for gerontological purposes and, as such, for public health initiatives to improve functionality of the otherwise-healthy older adults. From a clinical perspective, such an exclusive definition of sarcopenia is of far less relevance. Health care professionals, including physicians, nurses, physiotherapists, occupational therapists, and dieticians, rarely meet any individuals who are not affected by chronic diseases. Muscle wasting in older patients, which is of major relevance for health care professionals, is almost always a combined effect of aging and disease (**Fig. 1**).

Although there is a lack of precise data on the prevalence of age-specific sarcopenia, there might be a significant number of older adults suffering from such muscle loss. Some experience, so far, does not support this assumption. For example, clinical trials of selective androgen receptor modulators given to old adults with sarcopenia who are free of disease have been difficult to perform. Thus, it could be assumed that only a minor fraction of older people with reduced muscle mass could be said to have sarcopenia in the mere age-specific respect.

FROM MASS TO FUNCTION

Accumulating data have indicated that muscle mass is not linearly related to muscle function.[55,56] Longitudinal observational studies, for example, the Health ABC Study, have shown that the indices of function are better predictors of adverse outcomes than muscle mass.[57,58] Against this background, a new area of scientific discussions emerged that focused on the question whether to include function in the definition of sarcopenia. Most epidemiologic studies and few intervention studies have used the muscle mass–based definition of sarcopenia. However, growing evidences indicate that muscle function, as assessed by gait speed for instance, can now be considered as a strong predictive prognosis factor of survival.[59] Regulatory bodies likely do not acknowledge changes in muscle mass alone as an index of successful treatment in the pursuit of managing sarcopenia.

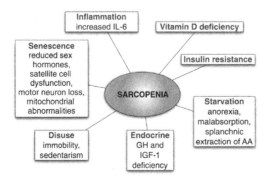

Fig. 1. The complex etiology of sarcopenia. AA, amino acid; GH, growth hormone; IGF-1, insulinlike growth factor 1; IL, interleukin.

NEW EFFORTS TO FIND A CLINICALLY RELEVANT DEFINITION OF SARCOPENIA

Scientists, mainly from the geriatric field, became concerned by the pending risk that the concept of sarcopenia could be lost for the clinical arena. It was claimed that a wider definition of sarcopenia was needed to make the concept clinically feasible. From around 2005 onward, several efforts were launched with the intention to come up with a clinically applicable definition (**Table 1**).

The major issues discussed have been the relevance of age, disease, and function in the context of sarcopenia; should anybody, irrespective of age, with reduced muscle mass, and irrespective of cause, be defined as having sarcopenia; and should function be involved in the definition.

The European Society of Parenteral and Enteral Nutrition Special Interest Groups Effort

In 2006, the European Society of Parenteral and Enteral Nutrition (ESPEN) Special Interest Group (SIG) of Nutrition in Geriatrics was established. This group gradually undertook the task to initiate a discussion on sarcopenia with stakeholders in the field. In a 3-day meeting of the BANSS Foundation in Germany in 2007, the subject was thoroughly considered. No consensus was reached, but the discussions were constructive and the controversies outlined. In parallel, the ESPEN SIG for Cachexia and Anorexia in Chronic Diseases was working on a document to refine the definition of cachexia with the intention to launch a precachexia definition. The 2 efforts were merged and the 2 SIGs presented a joined manuscript that was causing some turbulence but was finally published in 2010.[60] This document stated that, "sarcopenia is a condition characterized by loss of muscle mass and muscle strength. Although sarcopenia is primarily a disease of the elderly, its development may be associated with conditions that are not exclusively seen in older persons, like disuse, malnutrition and cachexia. Like osteopenia, it can also be seen in younger patients such as those with inflammatory diseases. The loss of muscle mass and muscle strength caused by such conditions is usually functionally less relevant in younger individuals, as their muscle mass and muscle strength is higher before it is affected by these conditions." The diagnosis was suggested to be based on the combined presence of a low muscle mass, that is, more than 2 SDs below the mean measured in young adults[53] and low gait speed of 0.8 m/s or less in a 4-meter walk test.[61]

The European Working Group on Sarcopenia in Older People

The European Union Geriatric Medicine Society (EUGMS) initiated a congregation of representatives from the EUGMS, the ESPEN, the International Association of Gerontology and Geriatrics—European Region, and the International Academy of Nutrition and Aging in the late 2008. During 2009, three 1- to 2-day seminars were organized, funded by the Abbott Laboratories, which resulted in a widely endorsed declaration.[62] Parts of this declaration were based on the newly introduced concept of sarcopenia being a geriatric syndrome,[63] describing a clinical condition in older persons, which is highly prevalent, multifactorial, and associated with poor outcomes. The wording of the agreed-on working definition is as follows, "Sarcopenia is a syndrome characterized by progressive and generalized loss of skeletal muscle mass and strength with a risk of adverse outcomes such as physical disability, poor quality of life and death." The diagnosis should be based on a documented reduced muscle mass (by DXA or BIA), for example, a T score of 2 SDs or more below mean in a young reference population plus at least 1 measure of reduced physical performance or muscle strength. Low physical performance could be gait speed less than 0.8 m/s[61] or a reduced score according

Table 1
Current efforts to define sarcopenia and suggested diagnostic criteria

Study Group	Definition	Criteria
The European Society of Parenteral and Enteral Nutrition Special Interest Groups	"Sarcopenia is a condition characterized by loss of muscle mass and muscle strength. Although sarcopenia is primarily a disease of the elderly, its development may be associated with conditions that are not exclusively seen in older persons, like disuse, malnutrition and cachexia. Like osteopenia, it can also be seen in younger patients such as those with inflammatory diseases"[60]	• Low muscle mass, eg, percentage of muscle mass >2 SDs below mean in individuals aged 18–39 y in the National Health and Nutrition Examination Survey III cohort • Walking speed <0.8 m/s in the 4-min test or reduced performance in any functional test used for the comprehensive geriatric assessment
The European Working Group on Sarcopenia in Older People	"Sarcopenia is a syndrome characterized by progressive and generalized loss of skeletal muscle mass and strength with a risk of adverse outcomes such as physical disability, poor quality of life and death."[62] The condition is called primary sarcopenia when the cause is aging per se and secondary sarcopenia when disease, inactivity, or malnutrition contribute	1. Low muscle mass 2. Low muscle strength, eg, grip strength 3. Low physical performance, eg, gait speed Reference population of healthy young subjects using cutoff points <2 SDs below mean. Criterion 1 and criterion 2 or 3
The International Working Group on Sarcopenia	"Sarcopenia is defined as the age-associated loss of skeletal muscle mass and function. The causes of sarcopenia are multi-factorial and can include disuse, altered endocrine function, chronic diseases, inflammation, insulin resistance, and nutritional deficiencies. While cachexia may be a component of sarcopenia, the two conditions are not the same"[65]	• Gait speed <1 m/s • Objectively measured low muscle mass, eg, appendicular mass relative to height squared, ie, ≤7.23 kg/m² in men and ≤5.67 kg/m² in women
The Society of Sarcopenia, Cachexia and Wasting Disorders	"Sarcopenia, ie, reduced muscle mass with limited mobility, is an important clinical entity and most older persons should be screened for this condition. The limitation in mobility should not clearly be due to otherwise defined specific diseases of muscle, peripheral vascular disease with intermittent claudication, central and peripheral nervous system disorders or cachexia" (Morley et al, personal communication, 2011)	• Walking speed ≤1 m/s or walking distance <400 m during a 6-min walk • A lean appendicular mass corrected for height squared of >2 SDs below the mean of healthy persons aged between 20 and 30 y of the same ethnic group
The Biomarkers Consortium	To be announced	To be announced

to the Short Physical Performance Battery, which combines gait speed, chair rising capacity and balance,[64] and reduced muscle strength, for example, grip strength or knee extension. Furthermore, an etiologic categorization was suggested, that is, primary sarcopenia when no cause other than aging was evident and secondary sarcopenia for activity-, disease-, and nutrition-related sarcopenia.[62] An algorithm for case finding was suggested to start with measuring gait speed in subjects at risk, and if the speed is low, the finding should be confirmed with muscle mass measurement. If the gait speed is normal, grip strength should be measured, and if the speed is reduced, the finding should be confirmed by muscle mass measurement.

The International Working Group on Sarcopenia

Based on the scientific network conferred by Gerontonet chaired by Professor Bruno Vellas, a group of geriatricians and scientists from academia and industry met in Rome, Italy, in November 2009 to reach a consensus definition of sarcopenia that could be shared by US and European Union stakeholders. The wording of the consensus is, "Sarcopenia is defined as the age-associated loss of skeletal muscle mass and function. The causes of sarcopenia are multi-factorial and can include disuse, altered endocrine function, chronic diseases, inflammation, insulin resistance, and nutritional deficiencies. While cachexia may be a component of sarcopenia, the two conditions are not the same. A diagnosis of sarcopenia is consistent with a gait speed of less than 1 m/s and an objectively measured low muscle mass, eg, appendicular muscle mass (DXA) relative to height squared that is ≤ 7.23 kg/m^2 in men and ≤ 5.67 kg/m^2 in women, ie, ≤ 20 percentile of values for healthy young adults."[65]

The Society of Sarcopenia, Cachexia and Wasting Disorders

After the introduction of the cachexia concept in 1997,[42] a new scene was set by the biannual Cachexia Conferences. During the first to fifth Cachexia Conferences, held between 2000 and 2009, discussions on muscle wasting during disease was a major issue.[66] These scientific efforts, meetings, and discussions were summoned during a consensus conference in 2006 and evolved into a well-accepted definition of cachexia that was published in 2008.[67] This definition outlined cachexia to be "a complex metabolic syndrome associated with underlying illness and characterized by loss of muscle with or without loss of fat mass. The prominent feature is weight loss. Anorexia, inflammation, insulin resistance and increased muscle protein breakdown are frequently associated with cachexia."

The organization around the Cachexia Meetings materialized into the formation of the Society of Sarcopenia, Cachexia and Wasting Disorders (SCWD). The SCWD has recently convened 2 expert panels. The first gave nutritional recommendations for the management of sarcopenia[68] and wrote, "at present, the definition of sarcopenia is evolving and the term sarcopenia is now often used to indicate the loss of muscle mass and function with chronic disease." A recent consensus conference on the definition of sarcopenia with representatives from the academy and industry, organized in Washington, DC, on December 2010, asserts that "sarcopenia, that is, reduced muscle mass with limited mobility, should be considered an important clinical entity and defined as a condition with muscle loss and reduced walking speed, that is, ≤ 1 m/s or a 6 minute walk of <400 m, and a T-score of lean appendicular mass corrected for height squared of ≤ 2SD" (Morley and colleagues, personal communication, 2011).

The Biomarkers Consortium Effort

In 2008, the National Institutes of Health (NIH) granted an initiative led by Professor Stephanie Studenski, including representatives of the NIH, the Food and Drug Administration, the pharmaceutical industry, and the research community. The goal was to come up with a definition of sarcopenia based on the answers to 2 questions: what is a clinically important degree of muscle wasting in older adults and, among older persons who are weak, what proportion demonstrates low muscle mass as a potentially treatable contributing cause. Six research groups have merged data from observational studies and clinical trials. "Phase II of this effort is to convene a consensus conference to review the analysis findings and create recommendations for the development of a consensus definition of sarcopenia and of the clinical criteria for its measurement acceptable to and useful for the purposes of all stakeholders" (citations from the NIH Web site, http://www.fnih.org/work/areas/life-stage/sarcopenia. Accessed May, 2011).[69]

SARCOPENIA BEYOND FUNCTION

The efforts so far have mainly focused on older persons and on options to widen the concept of sarcopenia with the aim to create a tool applicable in geriatric practice. Muscle tissue has functions other than locomotion alone. Cardiac output, respiratory integrity, glucose management and insulin sensitivity, drug tolerability, and amino acid supplies (especially in situations of metabolic stress) are examples of other important functions conferred by muscle tissue. Reduced muscle mass may display various adverse outcomes in patients with cancer, diabetes, chronic kidney disease, congestive heart failure, rheumatoid arthritis, and chronic obstructive pulmonary disease, to name only some disorders. It is likely, and it should also be encouraged, that the various etiologies of sarcopenia will call for separate definitions and, as a consequence, specific treatments in the future.

SUMMARY

The early concept of sarcopenia as a mere age-associated senescence-defined decline in muscle mass was productive for the purpose of investigating and understanding the role of age-specific pathogenic mechanisms of loss of muscle mass and function. For clinical purposes, a pure age-specific definition of sarcopenia is less fruitful. Most individuals, especially older persons, with reduced muscle mass and function display a mix of potential underlying mechanism, for example, chronic disease, nutritional deficiencies, and physical inactivity. There is no clear linearity between muscle mass and muscle function. Observational studies indicate that muscle function is a better predictor of clinical outcomes than muscle mass. This fact justifies function to be incorporated in the definition of sarcopenia.

Recently, 5 parallel initiatives have discussed adjustments of the definition of sarcopenia, mostly to increase the clinical usefulness of the definition. Three of the efforts are concluded, that is, those from the ESPEN SIGs of Nutrition in Geriatrics and Cachexia and Anorexia in Chronic Disease, the European Working Group on Sarcopenia in Older People, and the International Working Group on Sarcopenia. The pooled consensus, with some aberrations, is that sarcopenia is an important clinical entity, with multifactorial causes, such as senescence, chronic disease, physical inactivity, and poor food intake. Sarcopenia should be seen first and foremost, but not exclusively, as an age-related condition defined by the combined presence of reduced muscle mass, that is, a T score of muscle mass (corrected for height, body weight, or fat mass) of 2 SDs or less, and reduced muscle function measured as gait speed less than 0.8 or 1 m/s. The European Working Group also suggests the measurement of muscle strength, for example, grip strength or knee extension. With a clinically applicable definition, the ground is better laid for future clinical trials to amend the management of sarcopenia.

The evolving process of refining the definition of sarcopenia in accordance with the clinical needs and improved understanding of the complex etiology of this condition will continue.

REFERENCES

1. Rosenberg I. Summary comments: epidemiological and methodological problems in determining nutritional status of older persons. Am J Clin Nutr 1989;50:1231–3.
2. Christensen K, Doblhammer G, Rau R, et al. Ageing populations: the challenges ahead. Lancet 2009;374:1196–208.
3. United Nations. World population ageing: 1950–2050. Department of Economic and Social Affairs Population Division, DESA, United Nations: New York. 2006. Available at: http://www.un.org/esa/population/publications/worldageing19502050/. Accessed May, 2011.
4. Nair KS. Age-related changes in muscle. Mayo Clin Proc 2000;75(Suppl):S14–8.
5. Rosenberg IH. Sarcopenia: origins and clinical relevance. J Nutr 1997;127(Suppl 5): 990S–1S.
6. Evans WJ, Campbell WW. Sarcopenia and age-related changes in body composition and functional capacity. J Nutr 1993;123:465–8.
7. Holloszy J. Sarcopenia: muscle atrophy in old age. J Gerontol 1995;50A:1–161.
8. Evans W. What is sarcopenia? [Special issue]. J Gerontol 1995;50A:5–8.
9. Tzankoff SP, Norris AH. Longitudinal changes in basal metabolic rate in man. J Appl Physiol 1978;33:536–9.
10. Frontera WR, Hughes VA, Fielding RA, et al. Aging of skeletal muscle: a 12-yr longitudinal study. J Appl Physiol 2000;88(4):1321–6.
11. Ferrucci L, Guralnik JM, Buchner D, et al. Departures from linearity in the relationship between measures of muscular strength and physical performance of the lower extremities: the Women's Health and Aging Study. J Gerontol A Biol Sci Med Sci 1997;52:M275–85.
12. Cohn SH, Vartsky D, Yasumura S, et al. Compartmental body composition based on total-body nitrogen, potassium, and calcium. Am J Physiol 1980;239:E524–30.
13. Larsson L. Morphological and functional characteristics of the aging skeletal muscle in man. Acta Physiol Scand Suppl 1978;457(Suppl):1–36.
14. Larsson L. Histochemical characteristics of human skeletal muscle during aging. Acta Physiol Scand 1983;117:469–71.
15. Lexell J, Taylor CC, Sjostrom M. What is the cause of the ageing atrophy? Total number, size and proportion of different fiber types studied in whole vastus lateralis muscle from 15- to 83-year-old men. J Neurol Sci 1988;84:275–94.
16. Lexell J. Human aging, muscle mass, and fiber type composition. J Gerontol A Biol Sci Med Sci 1995;50(Spec No):11–6.
17. Marzetti E, Leeuwenburgh C. Skeletal muscle apoptosis, sarcopenia and frailty at old age. Exp Gerontol 2006;41:1234–8.
18. Edstrom E, Altun M, Bergman E, et al. Factors contributing to neuromuscular impairment and sarcopenia during aging. Physiol Behav 2007;92:129–35.
19. Doherty TJ, Vandervoort AA, Taylor AW, et al. Effects of motor unit losses on strength in older men and women. J Appl Physiol 1993;74:868–74.

20. Maggio M, Cappola AR, Ceda GP, et al. The hormonal pathway to frailty in older men. J Endocrinol Invest 2005;28(11 Suppl Proceedings):15–9.

21. Franceschi C, Capri M, Monti D, et al. Inflammaging and anti-inflammaging: a systemic perspective on aging and longevity emerged from studies in humans. Mech Ageing Dev 2007;128:92–105.

22. Schaap LA, Pluijm SM, Deeg DJ, et al. Inflammatory markers and loss of muscle mass (sarcopenia) and strength. Am J Med 2006;119:526.e9–526.e17.

23. Clavel S, Coldefy AS, Kurkdjian E, et al. Atrophy-related ubiquitin ligases, atrogin-1 and MuRF1 are up-regulated in aged rat tibialis anterior muscle. Mech Ageing Dev 2006;127:794–801.

24. Glass DJ. Signaling pathways perturbing muscle mass. Curr Opin Clin Nutr Metab Care 2010;13:225–9.

25. Glass D, Roubenoff R. Recent advances in the biology and therapy of muscle wasting. Ann N Y Acad Sci 2010;1211:25–36.

26. Short KR, Nair KS. The effect of age on protein metabolism. Curr Opin Clin Nutr Metab Care 2000;3:39–44.

27. D'Antona G, Nisoli E. mTOR signaling as a target of amino acid treatment of the age-related sarcopenia. Mobbs CV, Hof PR, editors. Body Composition and Aging; Karger: Basel (Switzerland). Interdiscip Top Gerontol 2010;37:115–41.

28. Thornell LE. Sarcopenic obesity: satellite cells in the aging muscle. Curr Opin Clin Nutr Metab Care 2010;14:22–7.

29. Liu W, Thomas SG, Asa SL, et al. Myostatin is a skeletal muscle target of growth hormone anabolic action. J Clin Endocrinol Metab 2003;88:5490–6.

30. Lang T, Cauley JA, Tylavsky F, et al. Computed tomography measurements of thigh muscle cross-sectional area and attenuation coefficient predict hip fracture: the Health, Aging and Body Composition Study. J Bone Miner Res 2010;25:513–9.

31. Guillet C, Boirie Y. Insulin resistance: a contributing factor to age-related muscle mass loss? Diabete Metab 2005;31(Spec No 2). 5S20–5S6.

32. Guillet C, Delcourt I, Rance M, et al. Changes in basal and insulin and amino acid response of whole body and skeletal muscle proteins in obese men. J Clin Endocrinol Metab 2009;94(8):3044–50.

33. Zamboni M, Mazzali G, Fantin F, et al. Sarcopenic obesity: a new category of obesity in the elderly. Nutr Metab Cardiovasc Dis 2008;18:388–95.

34. Moldawer LL, Copeland EM 3rd. Proinflammatory cytokines, nutritional support, and the cachexia syndrome: interactions and therapeutic options. Cancer 1997; 79:1828–39.

35. Argilés JM, López-Soriano FJ. The role of cytokines in cancer cachexia. Med Res Rev 1999;19:223–48.

36. Cederholm T, Wretlind B, Hellström K, et al. Enhanced generation of interleukins 1β and 6 may contribute to the cachexia of chronic disease. Am J Clin Nutr 1997; 65:876–82.

37. Pouw EM, Schols AM, Deutz NE, et al. Plasma and muscle amino acid levels in relation to resting energy expenditure and inflammation in stable chronic obstructive pulmonary disease. Am J Respir Crit Care Med 1998;158:797–801.

38. Stenvinkel P, Heimbürger O, Lindholm B, et al. Are there two types of malnutrition in chronic renal failure? Evidence for relationships between malnutrition, inflammation and atherosclerosis (MIA syndrome). Nephrol Dial Transplant 2000;15:953–60.

39. Baracos V, Rodemann HP, Dinarello CA, et al. Stimulation of muscle protein degradation and prostaglandin E2 release by leukocytic pyrogen (interleukin-1). A mechanism for the increased degradation of muscle proteins during fever. N Engl J Med 1983;308:553–8.

40. Cederholm T, Hellström K. Reversibility of protein-energy malnutrition in a group of chronically ill elderly out-patients. Clin Nutr 1995;14:81–7.

41. Creutzberg EC, Schols AM, Weling-Scheepers CA, et al. Characterization of non-response to high caloric oral nutritional therapy in depleted patients with chronic obstructive pulmonary disease. Am J Respir Crit Care Med 2000;161:745–52.

42. Roubenoff R, Heymsfield S, Kehayias J, et al. Standardization of nomenclature of body composition in weight loss. Am J Clin Nutr 1997;66:192–6.

43. Schols A, Buurman W, Staal van den Brekel A, et al. Evidence for a relation between metabolic derangements and increased levels of inflammatory mediators in a subgroup of patients with chronic obstructive pulmonary disease. Thorax 1996;51:819–24.

44. Anker SD, Ponikowski PP, Clark AL, et al. Cytokines and neurohormones relating to body composition alterations in the wasting syndrome of chronic heart failure. Eur Heart J 1999;20:683–93.

45. Baracos VE. Management of muscle wasting in cancer-associated cachexia: understanding gained from experimental studies. Cancer 2001;92(Suppl 6):1669–77.

46. Visser M, Pahor M, Taaffe DR, et al. Relationship of interleukin-6 and tumor necrosis factor-alpha with muscle mass and muscle strength in elderly men and women: the Health ABC Study. J Gerontol A Biol Sci Med Sci 2002;57:M326–32.

47. Biolo G, Bosutti A, Iscra F, et al. Contribution of the ubiquitin-proteasome pathway to overall muscle proteolysis in hypercatabolic patients. Metabolism 2000;49:689–91.

48. Baumgartner RN, Koehler KM, Gallagher D, et al. Epidemiology of sarcopenia among the elderly in New Mexico. Am J Epidemiol 1998;147(8):755–63.

49. Baumgartner RN, Waters DL, Gallagher D, et al. Predictors of skeletal muscle mass in elderly men and women. Mech Ageing Dev 1999;107:123–36.

50. Morley JE, Baumgartner RN, Roubenoff R, et al. Sarcopenia. J Lab Clin Med 2001;137:231–43.

51. Janssen I, Heymsfield SB, Ross R. Low relative skeletal muscle mass (sarcopenia) in older persons is associated with functional impairment and physical disability. J Am Geriatr Soc 2002;50:889–96.

52. Janssen I, Heymsfield SB, Baumgartner RN, et al. Estimation of skeletal muscle mass by bioelectrical impedance analysis. J Appl Physiol 2000;89:465–71.

53. Janssen I, Baumgartner RN, Ross R, et al. Skeletal muscle cutpoints associated with elevated physical disability risk in older men and women. Am J Epidemiol 2004;159:413–21.

54. Newman AB, Kupelian V, Visser M, et al. Sarcopenia: alternative definitions and associations with lower extremity function. J Am Geriatr Soc 2003;51:1602–9.

55. Visser M, Newman AB, Nevitt MC, et al. Reexamining the sarcopenia hypothesis. Muscle mass versus muscle strength. Ann N Y Acad Sci 2000;904:456–61.

56. Goodpaster BH, Carlson CL, Visser M, et al. Attenuation of skeletal muscle and strength in the elderly: the Health ABC Study. J Appl Physiol 2001;90:2157–65.

57. Visser M, Deeg DJ, Lips P, et al. Skeletal muscle mass and muscle strength in relation to lower-extremity performance in older men and women. J Am Geriatr Soc 2000;48:381–6.

58. Newman AB, Kupelian V, Visser M, et al. Strength, but not muscle mass, is associated with mortality in the health, aging and body composition study cohort. J Gerontol A Biol Sci Med Sci 2006;61:72–7.

59. Studenski S, Perera S, Patel K, et al. Gait speed and survival in older adults. JAMA 2011;305:50–8.

60. Muscaritoli M, Anker SD, Argiles J, et al. Consensus definition of sarcopenia, cachexia and pre-cachexia: joint document elaborated by Special Interest Groups (SIG) "cachexia-anorexia in chronic wasting diseases" and "nutrition in geriatrics". Clin Nutr 2010;29:154–9.

61. Guralnik JM, Ferrucci L, Pieper CF, et al. Lower extremity function and subsequent disability: consistency across studies, predictive models, and value of gait speed alone compared with the short physical performance battery. J Gerontol A Biol Sci Med Sci 2000;55:M221–31.

62. Cruz-Jentoft A, Baeyens JP, Bauer J, et al. Sarcopenia: European consensus on definition and diagnosis. Age Ageing 2010;39:412–23.

63. Cruz-Jentoft A, Landi F, Topinková E, et al. Understanding sarcopenia as a geriatric syndrome. Curr Opin Clin Nutr Metab Care 2010;13:1–7.

64. Guralnik JM, Simonsick EM, Ferrucci L, et al. A short physical performance battery assessing lower extremity function: association with self-reported disability and prediction of mortality and nursing home admission. J Gerontol 1994;49:M85–94.

65. Fielding R, Vellas B, Evans W, et al. Sarcopenia: an undiagnosed condition in older adults. Current consensus definition: prevalence, etiology, and consequences. International Working Group on Sarcopenia. J Am Med Dir Assoc 2011;12:249–56.

66. Morley JE, Anker SD, Evans WJ. Cachexia and aging: an update based on the fourth international cachexia meeting. J Nutr Health Aging 2009;13:47–55.

67. Evans WJ, Morley JE, Argiles J, et al. Cachexia: a new definition. Clin Nutr 2008; 27:793–9.

68. Morley JE, Argiles JM, Evans WJ, et al. Nutritional recommendations for the management of sarcopenia. J Am Med Dir Assoc 2010;11:391–6.

69. Available at: http://www.fnih.org/work/areas/life-stage/sarcopenia. Accessed May, 2011.

The Epidemiology of Sarcopenia

Ian Janssen, PhD

KEYWORDS

• Sarcopenia • Aged • Skeletal muscle • Elderly

One of the most dramatic age-related anatomic changes is that which occurs to skeletal muscle mass. In 1989, Rosenberg[1] coined the term sarcopenia to refer to the age-related loss in skeletal muscle mass and size. The term sarcopenia is derived from the Greek words *sarx* (flesh) and *penia* (loss). Rosenberg's rationale for creating a medical term to encapsulate age-related muscle loss was to bring increased awareness and attention to this process, which was not well understood or studied at that time. Consistent with Rosenberg's premise, the coining of the term sarcopenia led to a substantial increase in the research on the process, causes, consequences, and treatment of age-related muscle loss in the 1990s. This research focus has continued to the present time.

Several mechanisms are involved in the development of sarcopenia, including alterations in sex hormones, protein synthesis, proteolysis, neuromuscular integrity, endocrine issues (eg, insulin resistance), an increase in muscle fat content, changes in physical activity, and inadequate nutrition. An explanation of these mechanisms is beyond the scope of this review, and the reader is referred to other articles for a thorough discussion.[2–4] What is important to note here is that the mechanisms and causes of sarcopenia can vary from person to person. Recently, it has been suggested that primary sarcopenia be used to define sarcopenia that is caused by aging itself and that secondary sarcopenia be used to define sarcopenia that is caused by disuse (immobility, physical inactivity, or prolonged bed rest), disease (associated with advanced organ failure, inflammatory disease, malignancy, or endocrine disease), and/or inadequate nutrition and malabsorption (inadequate dietary intake of energy or protein, malabsorption, gastrointestinal disorders, or use of medications that cause anorexia).[5] In some individuals, a single cause of sarcopenia can be easily identified, whereas in others, there is no apparent single cause. Thus, it can be difficult or impossible to disentangle primary sarcopenia from secondary sarcopenia in a given older person.

The author is supported by an Early Researcher Award from the Ontario Ministry of Research and Innovation and a Tier 2 Canada Research Chair.
Conflicts of Interest: The author has nothing to disclose.
School of Kinesiology and Health Studies, Department of Community Health and Epidemiology, Queen's University, 28 Division Street, Kingston, ON K7L 3N6, Canada
E-mail address: Ian.janssen@queensu.ca

Clin Geriatr Med 27 (2011) 355–363
doi:10.1016/j.cger.2011.03.004

The findings from several longitudinal studies indicate that muscle mass and size decrease by approximately 6% per decade in the average person beginning at approximately 45 years of age.[6] Therefore, a typical 85-year-old person will have a muscle mass that is three-quarters of that when he or she was 45 years old. Even older adults who are active and healthy are not immune to the sarcopenia process, and it seems as though everybody loses muscle mass as they get older.[6] Thus, according to the definition originally proposed by Rosenberg, the prevalence of sarcopenia in the older adult population is 100%. With that being said, there are considerable differences from person to person in peak muscle mass (eg, muscle mass at approximately 25 years), the age at which muscle loss begins (eg, process may start at 40 years in a person and 50 years in another), and the amount of muscle that is lost over time. Because of these differences, there is a tremendous variation in the muscle mass values of older persons. Some older adults have a muscle mass that is comparable to that of healthy young adults, whereas other older adults have a muscle mass that is so low that their functional abilities and metabolic capacity may be severely compromised.

In 1998, Baumgartner and colleagues[7] proposed an alternative approach for identifying individuals with sarcopenia. Rather than defining sarcopenia as a process that all older persons go through, Baumgartner and colleagues proposed that an operational threshold be used to identify older persons who have healthy muscle mass values and those who have unhealthy muscle mass values, the latter they labeled as sarcopenic. More specifically, sarcopenia was defined as a height-adjusted appendicular muscle mass (arm + leg muscle mass/height^2) of 2 standard deviations or more below the mean of a young adult reference population. In that study, appendicular muscle mass was estimated using dual-energy x-ray absorptiometry (DXA). This approach for muscle is similar to how osteoporosis is defined and identified based on DXA bone density measurements.

As discussed below, the use of a threshold for identifying individuals with sarcopenia has proved to be particularly useful for epidemiologic research studies examining the prevalence of sarcopenia and the effect of sarcopenia on a variety of health outcomes. In addition to the thresholds originally proposed by Baumgartner and colleagues, several other threshold approaches have been used in the literature to identify individuals with sarcopenia. Some of these approaches are listed here:

- Whole-body muscle mass (kg) 2 standard deviations or more below the young adult mean. Muscle mass estimated using bioelectrical impedance analysis.[8]
- Whole-body muscle mass, expressed as a percentage of body weight, 2 standard deviations or more below the young adult mean. Muscle mass estimated using bioelectrical impedance analysis.[9]
- Lowest sex-specific quartile (lowest 25%) of height-adjusted appendicular muscle mass (kg/m^2). Appendicular muscle mass estimated using DXA.[10,11]
- Lowest sex-specific quartile of residuals obtained from a linear regression model wherein appendicular muscle mass was predicted from height and fat mass. Appendicular muscle mass estimated using DXA.[11]
- Lowest quartile of skeletal muscle area (cm^2) in mid-thigh. Skeletal muscle size estimated by computed tomography.[12,13]
- Height-adjusted whole-body muscle mass (kg/m^2) thresholds developed based on the relation between muscle mass and disability. Muscle mass estimated using bioelectrical impedance analysis.[14,15] This approach is conceptually different from all the other approaches listed above because it is based on the outcome and not the distribution of muscle within a population group.

PREVALENCE OF SARCOPENIA

The prevalence of sarcopenia observed in different research studies varies considerably. This reflects differences in the older population groups studied, the different techniques used to measure skeletal muscle mass and size, and differences in the normative (young and healthy) population groups that were used to derive the sarcopenia thresholds. Within the existing literature, the prevalence of sarcopenia in 60- to 70-year olds is in the order of 5% to 13%.[16] These prevalence estimates increase to 11% to 50% for the population aged 80 years or older.[16] Estimates for the World Health Organization[17] suggest that there were 600 million people aged 60 years or older in the year 2000 and that the number will increase to 1.2 billion by the year 2025. Conservative estimates based on the prevalence of sarcopenia and the World Health Organization population counts suggest that sarcopenia affects more than 50 million people today and that it will affect more than 200 million people over the next 40 years.[5]

INFLUENCE OF SARCOPENIA ON PHYSICAL FUNCTION

Most research on the health implications of sarcopenia that were published before 2005 focused on physical function outcomes, such as difficulty performing activity of daily living and instrumental activities of daily living.[6] The results from a few of the many cross-sectional studies are referred to in this paragraph to highlight the relationships that were reported. Using a cutoff for height-adjusted appendicular muscle mass of 2 standard deviations or more below the mean of young adults to define sarcopenia, Baumgartner and colleagues[7] reported that the likelihood of having physical disability was approximately 4 times greater in sarcopenic older men and women than in older persons with a normal muscle mass. In the Health Aging and Body Composition study, older adults in the lowest skeletal muscle quintile (adjusted for height and fat mass) were 80% to 90% more likely to have mobility impairment than older adults in the highest quintile.[11] Finally, in the US National Health and Nutrition Examination Survey, the likelihood of functional impairment and physical disability was 2- to 3-fold higher in older adults with severe sarcopenia than in older adults with a normal muscle mass.[9] In that study, severe sarcopenia was defined as a whole-body muscle mass, expressed as a percentage of body mass, less than 2 standard deviations below the mean of young adults. In summary, regardless of the approach used to identify a sarcopenic muscle mass, the associations between sarcopenia and physical function in these cross-sectional studies were moderate to strong in magnitude.

Because of the lack of temporality, these early cross-sectional studies cannot infer causation about the relationship between sarcopenia and physical function. Did a low muscle mass lead to functional impairment and disability, or did functional impairment and disability result in a lack of stimulation to muscle and muscle wasting? Both options are plausible. Longitudinal findings from prospective cohort studies that have been published in the past 5 or 6 years provide a stronger form of epidemiologic evidence on the cause and effect relationship between sarcopenia and physical function than what were previously available from the cross-sectional studies referred to above. Two published reports on the Health Aging and Body Composition cohort indicate that muscle size in the mid-thigh, as measured by computed tomography, was a weak to modest predictor of a loss in physical function over a 2- to 3-year follow-up.[12,13] In an 8-year follow-up of older adults from the Cardiovascular Health Study cohort, the risk of developing physical disability was 27% greater in those with severe sarcopenia than in those with a normal muscle mass.[14] In the same study, the likeli-hood of having physical disability at the start of the study (ie, baseline examination) was 79% greater in those with severe sarcopenia than in those with a normal muscle mass. Thus, the effect of sarcopenia on disability risk in the Cardiovascular Health Study was 3 times smaller in the longitudinal analysis than in the cross-sectional analysis. Taken together, the findings from these and other recent longitudinal studies imply that the effects of sarcopenia on functional impairment and physical disability inferred from the cross-sectional studies published in the late 1990s and early 2000s were significantly overestimated.

INFLUENCE OF SARCOPENIA ON METABOLIC FUNCTION, CHRONIC DISEASE, AND MORTALITY

Several recent studies have considered the effect of a low muscle mass on metabolic function, chronic disease, and mortality. One of the metabolic effects of a loss in muscle mass is a modest decrease in resting metabolic rate consequent to the loss in skeletal muscle mass.[18] Although it has been postulated that sarcopenia contrib-utes to metabolic and cardiovascular diseases, such as insulin resistance, type 2 dia-betes, dyslipidemia, and hypertension,[19] the literature is mixed and, in general, does not support this postulation. For instance, a study of 22 obese postmenopausal women found that those with sarcopenia, based on DXA measures of fat-free mass, had a more favorable lipid and lipoprotein profile than those without sarcopenia.[20] Additional research on more than 3000 members of the Cardiovascular Health Study cohort found that sarcopenia, as assed by whole-body measures of muscle mass that were estimated by bioelectrical impedance analysis, was not a risk factor for the development of cardiovascular disease over an 8-year follow-up period.[21]

A 2006 study reported that older patients with sarcopenia were twice as likely to contract infection during a hospital stay than were older patients with a normal muscle mass.[22] This suggests that individuals with sarcopenia may have a decreased immunity, which may provide a mechanistic link between sarcopenia and mortality risk, as observed in several studies. More specifically, studies of community dwelling[23,24] and institutionalized[25] older adults have shown that an upper-arm circumference measure, a crude index of sarcopenia, is predictive of both short-term and long-term mortality risk. Despite the consistency of observa-tions made in studies of upper-arm circumference, a study that relied on more precise measures of muscle mass obtained from computed tomography and DXA suggests that sarcopenia is a poor and clinically insignificant predictor of mortality risk in older adults.[26] Thus, it remains debatable as to whether sarcope-nia, defined based on the measures of muscle mass and size, is a risk factor for mortality.

RELEVANCE OF MUSCLE STRENGTH

A primary rationale for studying the age-related loss in muscle mass is the belief that the loss in muscle mass is indicative of a loss of muscle strength and function. Thus, in the causal chain, sarcopenia was thought to cause a loss in muscle strength, which in turn would cause functional impairment and physical disability. In fact, although the initial 1989 definition of sarcopenia focused exclusively on the loss in muscle mass, over time the definition of sarcopenia evolved into one that included both a loss in muscle mass and a loss in muscle strength and function. This evolved definition of sarcopenia can be seen in several literature reviews that were published around the turn of the century.[2,3,27]

The link between muscle mass and strength is supported by cross-sectional studies. For instance, a study reported that approximately 35% of the variability in muscle strength in young adults is predicted by muscle size.[28] Another study of 200 men and women aged 45 to 78 years found that the statistical adjustment for muscle mass substantially reduced the age-related differences in strength that were observed in the cohort.[29] The findings of several recent longitudinal studies bring into question these cross-sectional observations, as reviewed elsewhere.[30] One study in particular demonstrated that, within a sample of 120 adults aged 46 to 78 years at the study baseline and who were followed up for more than 10 years, less than 5% of the change in strength was attributable to the corresponding change in muscle size.[31] Thus, these longitudinal findings suggest that there is a disassociation between age-related changes in muscle mass and strength. Furthermore, the mechanisms that account for age-related declines in muscle mass and strength are different.[30]

Because of the apparent disconnect between the age-related loss in muscle mass and the age-related loss in muscle strength, in 2008, Clark and Manini[30] suggested that a distinct terminology be used to refer to these 2 phenomena. Specifically, they suggested that the term sarcopenia be reserved to its initial definition of the age-related loss in muscle mass and that the term dynapenia be used to describe the age-related changes in muscle strength.[30] The Greek term dynapenia translates to poverty of strength.

There is evidence that dynapenia is a risk factor for functional impairment and physical disability.[12,13,32] Consider for instance the findings from the Health Aging Body Composition cohort.[13] The findings in question were based on 3075 well-functioning black and white men and women aged 70 to 79 years who were followed up for 2.5 years. In this study, muscle size in the mid-thigh was measured using computed tomography and knee extensor strength using a dynamometer. Men and women in the lowest muscle strength quartile had approximately double the risk of developing mobility limitations during the follow-up period than those in the highest muscle strength quartile. In addition to functional problems, there is evidence that dynapenia is a risk factor for other health outcomes. A series of published reports from the Aerobics Center Longitudinal Study have demonstrated that, by comparison with those in the lowest strength group (eg, top quartile), those in the highest strength group are 45% less likely to have the metabolic syndrome,[33] 39% less likely to die of cancer,[34] and 20% less likely to die of all causes.[35] Research also suggests that muscle strength is related to insulin resistance[36] and type 2 diabetes.[37]

An intriguing question is whether a low muscle mass (sarcopenia) or low muscle strength (dynapenia) is a stronger predictor of physical function, chronic disease, and mortality risk. The evidence consistently points toward strength as being the stronger predictor. Visser and colleagues[13] demonstrated that a low muscle mass and low muscle strength were risk factors for mobility decline in older men and women. However, although a low muscle strength remained an independent predictor of mobility decline after consideration of muscle mass, a low muscle mass was not a predictor of mobility decline after consideration of muscle strength.[13] Stephen and Janssen[21] have recently published findings indicating that dynapenic obesity, but not sarcopenic obesity, is a significant predictor of cardiovascular disease risk.[21] Newman and colleagues[26] reported that older individuals with dynapenia have a 50% increased all-cause mortality risk independent of sarcopenia but that individuals with sarcopenia do not have a significantly increased all-cause mortality risk independent of dynapenia. When coupled with the observation that losses in muscle strength are not directly attributable to age-related losses in muscle mass, these findings imply that research and clinical emphasis should be placed more on muscle strength and function than on muscle size.

CONSENSUS DEFINITION OF SARCOPENIA

The sarcopenia research that has been conducted over the past 2 decades has not been well integrated into clinical practice. Part of this reflects the vast array of definitions, thresholds, and measures that different researchers have used to identify the condition. To address this issue, the European Working Group on Sarcopenia in Older People (EWGSOP) was developed in 2009 to develop a consensus definition of sarcopenia that could be used in both the research and clinical settings. The EWGSOP included representatives from 4 organizations (European Geriatric Medicine Society, European Society for Clinical Nutrition and Metabolism, International Association of Gerontology and Geriatrics—European Region, and International Association of Nutrition and Aging), all of which endorsed the consensus definition and report that were produced by the EWGSOP.[5]

The EWGSOP consensus definition for sarcopenia is intended to be practical. It relies on 3 measures: low muscle mass, low muscle strength, and low physical performance. The consensus definition is based on a staging system that includes 3 stages: presarcopenia, sarcopenia, and severe sarcopenia. The presarcopenia stage is characterized by low muscle mass with a normal muscle strength and normal physical performance. The sarcopenia stage is characterized by a low muscle mass and either a low muscle strength or a low physical performance. The severe sarcopenia stage is characterized by the presence of all 3 criteria (low muscle mass, low muscle strength, and low physical performance).

To identify low muscle mass and low muscle strength, the EWGSOP recommends the use of normative (healthy young adult) reference populations, with 2 standard deviations below the mean of the normative population used as the threshold to identify a low muscle mass and low muscle strength. These thresholds depend on the availability of reference studies and the measurement technique chosen. For example, for muscle mass, DXA could be used to assess appendicular muscle mass[7,38,39] or bioelectrical impedance analysis to estimate whole-body muscle mass.[9,14,40] Likewise, muscle strength could be assessed using a simple measure such as handgrip strength (obtained on a handgrip dynamometer)[41,42] or a more complex measure such as knee extension strength (obtained using an isokinetic dynamometer).[38,43] The working group indicated that research is urgently needed to obtain good reference values for muscle mass and muscle strength for populations around the world.

A wide range of tests are available to assess a low physical performance. Although the EWGSOP did not make a specific recommendation as to which performance test be used for sarcopenia assessment, a special emphasis was placed in their report on usual gait speed and the Short Physical Performance Battery (SPPB). A cutoff point of 0.8 m/s or more for usual gait speed (over a 4- to 6-m course) was suggested as the threshold for poor performance in a walking speed test.[44] The SPPB evaluates balance, gait, strength, and endurance by examining an individual's ability to stand with the feet together in side-by-side, semi-tandem, and tandem positions; time to walk 8 ft; and time to rise from a chair and return to the seated position 5 times.[45] The balance, walking speed, and chair stand tests are given scores between 0 and 4, with a maximum total score of 12. SPPB scores of 8 or less can be used to denote poor physical performance.[45]

SUMMARY

Research conducted within the past 2 decades has taught us a considerable amount about the health consequences of the age-related loss in muscle mass and strength. Although there is a large body of epidemiologic evidence linking sarcopenia (particularly a low muscle strength) to a loss in physical function, cardiometabolic disease, and mortality, the assessment and management of sarcopenia are not a routine part of clinical practice. It is hoped that the development of a consensus and clinical-friendly definition of sarcopenia by the EWGSOP will help promote the recognition and treatment of age-related sarcopenia in the clinical setting.

REFERENCES

1. Rosenberg IR. Summary comments. Am J Clin Nutr 1989;50:1231–3.
2. Morley JE, Baumgartner RN, Roubenoff R, et al. Sarcopenia. J Lab Clin Med 2001;137(4):231–43.
3. Roubenoff R. Origins and clinical relevance of sarcopenia. Can J Appl Physiol 2001;26(1):78–89.
4. Rolland Y, Czerwinski S, Abellan Van Kan G, et al. Sarcopenia: its assessment, etiology, pathogenesis, consequences and future perspectives. J Nutr Health Aging 2008;12(7):433–50.
5. Cruz-Jentoft AJ, Baeyens JP, Bauer JM, et al. Sarcopenia: European consensus on definition and diagnosis: report of the European Working Group on Sarcopenia in Older People. Age Ageing 2010;39(4):412–23.
6. Janssen I, Ross R. Linking age-related changes in skeletal muscle mass and composition with metabolism and disease. J Nutr Health Aging 2005;9:408–19.
7. Baumgartner RN, Koehler KM, Gallagher D, et al. Epidemiology of sarcopenia among the elderly in New Mexico. Am J Epidemiol 1998;147(8):755–63.
8. Cruz-Jentoft AJ, Landi F, Topinkova E, et al. Understanding sarcopenia as a geriatric syndrome. Curr Opin Clin Nutr Metab Care 2010;13(1):1–7.
9. Janssen I, Heymsfield SB, Ross R. Low relative skeletal muscle mass (sarcopenia) in older persons is associated with functional impairment and physical disability. J Am Geriatr Soc 2002;50(5):889–96.
10. Delmonico MJ, Harris TB, Lee JS, et al. Alternative definitions of sarcopenia, lower extremity performance, and functional impairment with aging in older men and women. J Am Geriatr Soc 2007;55(5):769–74.
11. Newman AB, Kupelian V, Visser M, et al. Sarcopenia: alternative definitions and associations with lower extremity function. J Am Geriatr Soc 2003;51(11):1602–9.
12. Goodpaster BH, Park SW, Harris TB, et al. The loss of skeletal muscle strength, mass, and quality in older adults: the health, aging and body composition study. J Gerontol A Biol Sci Med Sci 2006;61(10):1059–64.
13. Visser M, Goodpaster BH, Kritchevsky SB, et al. Muscle mass, muscle strength, and muscle fat infiltration as predictors of incident mobility limitations in well-functioning older persons. J Gerontol A Biol Sci Med Sci 2005;60(3):324–33.
14. Janssen I. Influence of sarcopenia on the development of physical disability: the Cardiovascular Health Study. J Am Geriatr Soc 2006;54(1):56–62.
15. Janssen I, Baumgartner RN, Ross R, et al. Skeletal muscle cutpoints associated with elevated physical disability risk in older men and women. Am J Epidemiol 2004;159(4):413–21.
16. Morley JE. Sarcopenia: diagnosis and treatment. J Nutr Health Aging 2008;12(7): 452–6.

17. World Health Organization. Ageing and life course. Available at: http://www.who. int/ageing/en/. Accessed March 3, 2011.

18. Lammes E, Akner G. Resting metabolic rate in elderly nursing home patients with multiple diagnoses. J Nutr Health Aging 2006;10(4):263–70.

19. Karakelides H, Sreekumaran Nair K. Sarcopenia of aging and its metabolic impact. Curr Top Dev Biol 2005;68:123–48.

20. Aubertin-Leheudre M, Lord C, Goulet ED, et al. Effect of sarcopenia on cardio-vascular disease risk factors in obese postmenopausal women. Obesity (Silver Spring) 2006;14(12):2277–83.

21. Stephen WC, Janssen I. Sarcopenic-obesity and cardiovascular disease risk in the elderly. J Nutr Health Aging 2009;13(5):460–6.

22. Cosqueric G, Sebag A, Ducolombier C, et al. Sarcopenia is predictive of nosoco-mial infection in care of the elderly. Br J Nutr 2006;96(5):895–901.

23. Miller MD, Crotty M, Giles LC, et al. Corrected arm muscle area: an independent predictor of long-term mortality in community-dwelling older adults? J Am Geriatr Soc 2002;50(7):1272–7.

24. Prothro JW, Rosenbloom CA. Body measurements of black and white elderly persons with emphasis on body composition. Gerontology 1995;41(1):22–38.

25. Muhlethaler R, Stuck AE, Minder CE, et al. The prognostic significance of protein-energy malnutrition in geriatric patients. Age Ageing 1995;24(3):193–7.

26. Newman AB, Kupelian V, Visser M, et al. Strength, but not muscle mass, is asso-ciated with mortality in the health, aging and body composition study cohort. J Gerontol A Biol Sci Med Sci 2006;61(1):72–7.

27. Vandervoot AA, Symons TB. Functional and metabolic consequences of sarcope-nia. Can J Appl Physiol 2001;26(1):90–101.

28. Maughan RJ, Watson JS, Weir J. Strength and cross-sectional area of human skeletal muscle. J Physiol 1983;338(5):37–49.

29. Frontera WR, Hughes VA, Lutz KJ, et al. A cross-sectional study of muscle strength and mass in 45- to 78-yr-old men and women. J Appl Physiol 1991; 71(2):644–50.

30. Clark BC, Manini TM. Sarcopenia =/= dynapenia. J Gerontol A Biol Sci Med Sci 2008;63(8):829–34.

31. Hughes VA, Frontera WR, Wood M, et al. Longitudinal muscle strength changes in older adults: influence of muscle mass, physical activity, and health. J Gerontol A Biol Sci Med Sci 2001;56(5):B209–17.

32. Carmeli E, Reznick AZ, Coleman R, et al. Muscle strength and mass of lower extremities in relation to functional abilities in elderly adults. Gerontology 2000; 46(5):249–57.

33. Jurca R, Lamonte MJ, Barlow CE, et al. Association of muscular strength with inci-dence of metabolic syndrome in men. Med Sci Sports Exerc 2005;37(11):1849–55.

34. Ruiz JR, Sui X, Lobelo F, et al. Muscular strength and adiposity as predictors of adulthood cancer mortality in men. Cancer Epidemiol Biomarkers Prev 2009; 18(5):1468–76.

35. FitzGerald SJ, Barlow CE, Kampert JB, et al. Muscular fitness and all-cause mortality: prospective observations. J Phys Act Health 2004;1(1):7–18.

36. Karelis AD, Tousignant B, Nantel J, et al. Association of insulin sensitivity and muscle strength in overweight and obese sedentary postmenopausal women. Appl Physiol Nutr Metab 2007;32(2):297–301.

37. Sayer AA, Dennison EM, Syddall HE, et al. Type 2 diabetes, muscle strength, and impaired physical function: the tip of the iceberg? Diabetes Care 2005;28(10): 2541–2.

38. Bouchard DR, Heroux M, Janssen I. Association between muscle mass, leg strength, and fat mass with physical function in older adults: influence of age and sex. J Aging Health 2011;23(2):313–28.
39. Baumgartner RN. Body composition in healthy aging. Ann N Y Acad Sci 2000; 904:437–48.
40. Janssen I, Heymsfield SB, Baumgartner RN, et al. Estimation of skeletal muscle mass by bioelectrical impedance analysis. J Appl Physiol 2000;89(2):465–71.
41. Rantanen T, Harris T, Leveille SG, et al. Muscle strength and body mass index as long-term predictors of mortality in initially healthy men. J Gerontol A Biol Sci Med Sci 2000;55(3):M168–73.
42. Rantanen T, Guralnik JM, Foley D, et al. Midlife hand grip strength as a predictor of old age disability. JAMA 1999;281(6):558–60.
43. Rantanen T, Guralnik JM, Sakari-Rantala R, et al. Disability, physical activity, and muscle strength in older women: the Women's Health and Aging Study. Arch Phys Med Rehabil 1999;80(2):130–5.
44. Working Group on Functional Outcome Measures for Clinical Trials. Functional outcomes for clinical trials in frail older persons: time to be moving. J Gerontol A Biol Sci Med Sci 2008;63(2):160–4.
45. Guralnik JM, Simonsick EM, Ferrucci L, et al. A short physical performance battery assessing lower extremity function: association with self-reported disability and prediction of mortality and nursing home admission. J Gerontol 1994;49(2):M85–94.

Physiopathological Mechanism of Sarcopenia

Stéphane Walrand, PhD[a,b], Christelle Guillet, PhD[a,b],
Jérome Salles, PhD[a,b], Noël Cano, MD, PhD[a,b,c],
Yves Boirie, MD, PhD[a,b,c],*

KEYWORDS

• Sarcopenia • Nutrition • Exercise • Hormones

Muscle erosion, which begins after the age of 55 years, is one of the most important factors of disability in elderly people. The cumulative decline in muscle mass reaches 40% from 20 to 80 years. The magnitude of this phenomenon, termed "sarcopenia," as a public health problem is not well established because there are few epidemiologic and longitudinal studies focusing on the decrements of strength and muscle mass with advancing age. However, it is estimated that the direct health care cost attributable to sarcopenia in the United States in 2000 was $18.5 billion, which represented about 1.5% of total health care expenditures for that year.[1] The reduction in muscle mass and strength provokes an impaired mobility and increased risk for falls and fall-related fractures. In addition, muscle loss is associated with a decrease in overall physical activity levels with subsequent metabolic alterations, such as obesity, insulin resistance, and a reduction in bone density in the elderly. As the elderly population increases around the world, the involuntary loss of muscle mass with aging may become a major health problem in the years to come. Sedentary individuals, subjects with poor protein intake, and those suffering from debilitating diseases are also at greater risks of sarcopenia.

Sarcopenia is believed to be caused predominantly by atrophy and loss of skeletal muscle fibers, mainly type II fibers. This results in a relative elevation in type I fiber density related to a supposed preservation of muscle endurance and a reduction in muscle strength. Biochemically, muscle size, function, and composition are closely regulated by muscle protein turnover. Consequently, the age-related loss of muscle

[a] INRA, UMR 1019, UNH, CRNH Auvergne, Clermont-Ferrand, F-63009, France
[b] Université Clermont 1, UFR de Médecine, UMR 1019, UNH, Clermont-Ferrand, F-63001, France
[c] Service de Nutrition Clinique, CHU Clermont-Ferrand, Hôpital Gabriel Montpied, Clermont-Ferrand, F-63003, France
* Corresponding author. Laboratoire de Nutrition Humaine, 58 rue Montalembert, BP321, 63009 Clermont-Ferrand cedex 1, France.
E-mail address: boirie@clermont.inra.fr

Clin Geriatr Med 27 (2011) 365–385
doi:10.1016/j.cger.2011.03.005   **geriatric.theclinics.com**
0749-0690/11/$ – see front matter © 2011 Elsevier Inc. All rights reserved.

proteins results from an imbalance between protein synthesis and degradation rates. Until now, most reports have indicated that muscle protein synthesis declines with age. The studies have demonstrated that synthesis rates of various muscle fractions, such as myofibrillar and mitochondrial fractions, decline in the elderly or even by middle age. Reduced protein turnover adversely affects muscle function by inducing protein loss and damaged protein accumulation. Data also suggest that sarcopenia is cause by failure of muscle protein synthesis in the postabsorptive and the fed state. Other factors, such as neurodegenerative processes with loss of alpha motor neurons in the spinal column, dysregulation of anabolic hormone (insulin, growth, and sex hormones) and cytokine productions, modification in the response to inflammatory events, inadequate nutritional intake, and sedentarity may also participate in muscle loss during aging. The determinants of sarcopenia include genetic and environmental factors, with a complex series of poorly understood interactions. It is still unknown whether muscle loss of aged people is an inevitable condition of aging per se, or if illnesses, inappropriate nutrition, sedentarity, and other lifestyle habits are the major causes of sarcopenia. Currently, because the pathophysiology of sarcopenia is poorly understood, nutritional interventions either to prevent or at least to limit this condition are extremely limited.[2]

MECHANISMS OF SARCOPENIA

Many explanations for muscle decline in elderly people have been proposed. Those mechanisms that are eventually preventable or modified are discussed with a special emphasis on nutritional aspects.

Age-Related Changes in Hormone Levels and Sensitivity

Aging is associated with modifications of hormone production and sensitivity especially with regard to growth hormone (GH), insulin-like growth factor (IGF)-I, corticosteroids, androgens, estrogens, and insulin. These hormones may influence the anabolic and catabolic state for an optimal muscle protein metabolism. A decrease in GH and IGF-I levels is frequently demonstrated in elderly people[3] and this is paralleled by changes in body composition (ie, increased visceral fat and decreased lean body mass and bone mineral density). It was tempting to treat patients suffering from muscle loss by GH injections, but no evidence of increased muscle strength was reported even if an increased muscle mass may occur.[4,5]

Similar changes in body composition are seen in the state of hypercortisolism so that cortisol/GH ratio has been proposed as an important factor for changes in body composition.[6] Increasing age can be associated with elevated evening cortisol levels in men but changes in the sensitivity of the hypothalamic-pituitary-adrenal axis also occur with increasing age, resulting in an age-related decline in the resilience of the hypothalamic-pituitary-adrenal axis. This might lead to an increased exposure of several tissues to glucocorticoids with aging.

Aging is associated with low testosterone, which may lead to decreased muscle mass and bone strength, and thereby to more fractures and complications. Some intervention studies are ongoing to counteract muscle loss related to chronic diseases with some promising results.

Finally, the impact of insulin resistance on age-related muscle loss has been recently proposed because it is well known that increase in intramyocellular fat mass is associated with an increased risk of insulin resistance with aging. A decreased response to insulin was demonstrated as the result of an impaired insulin signaling or an impaired insulin-mediated increased in muscle blood flow.[7]

Inflammation and Sarcopenia

Proinflammatory cytokines (tumor necrosis factor [TNF]-α, interleukin [IL]-1β and -6) promote muscle wasting directly by increasing myofibrillar protein degradation[8] and by decreasing protein synthesis.[9] Enhancement of proteolysis is accomplished by activation of the ubiquitin-dependent proteolytic system[10] because TNF-α activates several serine and threonine kinases and intracellular factors, including the inhibitor of the nuclear factor-kappa B (NFκB [IκB]). IL-6 is also involved in the regulation of muscle protein turnover and is considered to be a catabolic cytokine.[11] This activation contributes to trigger NF-κB, which is implicated in the upregulation of myofibrillar proteolysis by the proteasome system and in the suppression of myofibrillar protein synthesis. TNF-α impairs skeletal muscle protein synthesis by decreasing translational efficiency and initiation associated with alteration in the eukaryotic initiation factor (eIF)-4E. An indirect effect of TNF-α on muscle protein metabolism may also be its capacity to inhibit insulin action because this hormone has been shown to increase muscle protein synthesis and to decrease proteolysis.[12,13] It is now clear that many other inflammatory factors exhibit the same impact on muscle. Concerning protein metabolism, administration of leptin may result in a decreased rate of myofibrillar protein synthesis in skeletal muscle.[14] IL-6 and resistin are other well-characterized examples of compounds produced in adipose tissue that may participate in the regulation of muscle metabolism. Interestingly, the depletion of muscle mass with age does not necessarily result in weight loss, suggesting that a corresponding accumulation of body fat occurs. Abdominal fat accumulation with aging is another candidate for a low-grade inflammation process that may affect muscle protein metabolism and function. Indeed, aging is associated with increased levels of circulating inflammatory components in blood including elevated concentrations of TNF-α; IL-6; IL-1 receptor antagonist; soluble TNF receptor (sTNFR1); acute phase proteins, such as C-reactive protein; and high neutrophil counts.[15] This chronic low-grade inflammation is associated with a variety of pathologic phenomena that may affect the elderly, including sarcopenia, osteoporosis, atherosclerosis, reduced immune function, and insulin resistance.

IMPAIRED RESPONSE OF PROTEIN METABOLISM TO NUTRITION

Impaired Anabolic Response of Skeletal Muscle to Nutrition

Muscle loss in elderly subjects may depend on both inadequate nutritional intake and impaired adaptation of skeletal muscle to nutrients (eg, essential amino acids).[16] By using femoral arteriovenous catheterization and quadriceps muscle biopsies, Volpi and colleagues[17] have reported that a peripheral infusion of an amino acid mixture was able to increase amino acid delivery to the leg, amino acid transport, and muscle protein synthesis irrespective of age.[17] Despite no change in protein breakdown during amino acid infusion, a positive net balance of amino acids across the muscle was achieved. The authors concluded that, although muscle mass is decreased in the elderly, muscle protein anabolism can nonetheless be stimulated by a high amino acid availability.[17] The same observation was described with an oral administration of a large dose of amino acid mixture, but a higher first-pass splanchnic extraction of leucine and phenylalanine was demonstrated.[18,19] Amino acid transport into muscle, muscle protein synthesis, and net balance increased similarly in both the young and the elderly suggesting that muscle protein anabolism can be stimulated by oral amino acids in the elderly and in young subjects. Similarly, muscle protein synthesis increased to the same extent after an oral intake of either balanced amino acids or essential amino acids in the healthy elderly.[20] Therefore, even if nonessential amino acids seem not to be required to stimulate muscle protein anabolism in older adults, muscle response to nutrients, especially amino acid intake, is preserved in elderly subjects compared with younger subjects. However, the amount and the quality of dietary proteins and the energy added to protein intake are more important to consider. Indeed, when glucose was associated with an oral administration of a mixture of amino acids,[21] an increased amino acid delivery and transport into the muscle together with a decreased muscle protein breakdown was achieved. However, the stimulation of muscle protein synthesis in the young no more exists in the elderly subjects leading to a lower protein balance in the leg skeletal muscles. The anabolic response of muscle protein to hyperaminoacidemia and to higher levels of endogenous insulin seems to be impaired in the healthy elderly as a result of a blunted response of protein synthesis, implying that the route and the nonprotein substrates added to amino acids on net muscle protein anabolism in young and elderly subjects has to be taken into account.[18,21] These studies led us to open the question of muscle sensitivity to hormones, such as insulin, and the impact of normal or low protein intake during aging. Indeed, a previous study[22] has demonstrated in old rats that the anabolic response of muscle protein metabolism to a complete meal is blunted compared with young adult animals. This lack of muscle anabolic response to meal intake may contribute to the long-term development of sarcopenia in the elderly.

Protein Intake and Quality of Dietary Proteins to Counteract the Anabolic Resistance of Skeletal Muscle

Quantitative aspects

The mean dietary requirement for adult men and women of all ages, as set by the metaanalysis of Rand and colleagues,[23] was estimated to be 0.66 g protein/kg/d, with a suggested safe level of intake set at 0.83 g protein/kg/d.[23] However, because body composition and protein metabolism changes occur with age, especially related to muscle, it has been suggested that the use of dietary proteins and amino acids may differ between young and old adults. Consequently, using various methodologies (ie, nitrogen balance and tracer procedures), protein requirement with advancing age was discussed. Taken together, studies based on nitrogen balance using the same formula showed that protein requirement increases in elderly people. When the recalculated data from all studies were combined by weighted mean averages, a mean protein requirement of 0.89 g protein/kg/d was estimated.[24,25] Nevertheless, recent work based on tracer methodology reported that the rate of whole-body protein turnover, a commonly assumed determinant of protein requirement, exhibited nonsignificant change with age when expressed per kilogram of fat-free mass.[26,27] However, because of modification in body composition and physiologic function that occurs with the lower even above normal recommended daily allowance for proteins, protein requirement might be increased in healthy elderly people.[2] Nonetheless, in hospitalized patients calculations from spontaneous nitrogen intakes and loss indicated a safe protein intake of at least 1.3 g protein/kg/d.[28] Because nitrogen balance and tracer studies are still controversial, recommendations for protein intake in this population are still debated.

There is even less information about the upper limit for protein intake in older people. Very few experiments were designed to study the effect of increased or high protein intake in the elderly population. Whole-body protein turnover was enhanced in elderly men and women when the protein amount in the diet increased from 12% to 21% of total energy.[29] Walrand and colleagues[30] recently showed that a high-protein diet (ie, 3 g/kg fat free mass per day for 10 days) was inefficient to enhance protein synthesis at whole-body and skeletal muscle levels. Interestingly, in this study, although a high-protein diet enhanced glomerular filtration rate in young adults, it reduced renal function in the aged group, suggesting that a very high protein diet may be deleterious in healthy subjects.

Inversely, following a low protein intake (50% of usual intake), no modification of whole-body protein synthesis and breakdown was noticed in a group of aged women.[31] However, whole-body protein oxidation, nitrogen balance, muscle mass, muscle function, and immune responses were significantly affected in the group fed a low-protein diet.[32] Collectively, these observations highlight the importance of maintaining adequate protein intakes in elderly people to counteract the negative effect of aging on protein metabolism. The recently published Health ABC study clearly indicates that during a 3-year follow-up, elderly subjects consuming a higher amount of daily protein have a lesser reduction in appendicular lean body mass.[33]

Qualitative impact of dietary proteins during aging
It is possible that the impact on protein metabolism of the different types of dietary protein is not the same. The consumption of three different protein sources and their effect on protein metabolism was analyzed in elderly women.[34] A first diet was composed half of animal proteins and half of vegetable proteins, whereas one third of the proteins consumed in the second diet were from vegetable and two third from animals, and inversely in the third diet. Nitrogen balance was not modified in this study but whole-body protein breakdown was not inhibited to the same extent by the meal when the protein source was from vegetables compared with meat.[34] This study showed that intake of high-quality proteins may be an important issue in elderly people.

Another important consideration regarding the quality of dietary protein is the speed of protein absorption from the gut. By analogy with carbohydrates, protein can be digested at different rates (ie, concept of "fast" and "slow" proteins).[35] For example, the two main milk proteins, casein and whey protein, have different behaviors in the intestinal tract. Whey protein, a soluble protein, is considered as a fast protein: after digestion and absorption, plasma appearance of amino acids derived from this protein is high and fast, but transient. On the contrary, casein clots in the stomach, which delays its gastric emptying and therefore results in a slower, lower, but prolonged release and absorption of amino acids. This new concept was recently applied to the modification of protein metabolism during aging.[36] In this population, the duration and magnitude of elevated plasma amino acids are key factors to counteract the decrease in muscle sensitivity to amino acids. Accordingly, postprandial protein gain was higher after a meal containing fast protein (ie, whey protein) than slow protein (ie, casein) in elderly, when considering either isonitrogenous or isoleucine (because leucine is a well-known anabolic factor) meals. In addition, postprandial protein use by the body was significantly higher with the fast than with the slow protein.[36] A recent report[37] also showed that whey proteins are able to stimulate muscle protein synthesis rate in a group of healthy elderly individuals. These data clearly suggest that a protein mixture that can be quickly digested and absorbed might be more efficient to limit protein loss during aging than a mixture yielding slower kinetics.

Recent studies have determined the mechanism of decreased skeletal muscle sensitivity to amino acids in elderly people.[38] A defect in branched chain amino acid activation pathway may be responsible for this alteration. Consequently, the alteration of muscle protein synthesis response to anabolic signals may be counteracted by nutritional strategies aimed at improving branched chain amino acid availability. Within the dietary proteins, essential amino acids are very important for muscle anabolism. For example, in vitro or in vivo high leucine administration is able to stimulate muscle protein synthesis rate in aged rodents.[39-41] In these models, leucine acts as an actual mediator able to modulate specific intracellular pathways linked with the stimulation of protein translation.[42] Interestingly, when given to old rats for 10 days, the beneficial effect of leucine supplementation persisted, indicating that a long-term use of leucine-enriched diets may limit muscle wasting in aged individuals.[43] In addition, these data suggest that nutritional manipulation increasing the availability of leucine into skeletal muscle, such as the use of the leucine-rich fast protein (ie, whey protein), could be beneficial to improve postprandial protein retention during aging. The beneficial effect of such a diet on muscle protein synthesis in aged humans is currently under study.

Daily protein feeding pattern
The impact of daily protein distribution might be crucial for a better protein anabolism. Studies by Arnal and colleagues[44,45] clearly demonstrate that a protein feeding pattern that combines meals rich and low in proteins during the day may improve protein retention in elderly persons. A "spread" diet composed of four meals spreading daily protein intake over 12 hours was compared with a pulse diet providing 80% of daily protein intake concentrated at midday. The pulse protein pattern was more efficient at improving nitrogen balances and whole-body protein retention in aged people. The pulse protein diet possesses two advantages: the midday protein pulse meal may stimulate whole-body synthesis by highly increasing amino acid concentration, and high-carbohydrate and low-protein meals are known to limit protein loss by reducing protein breakdown rate via postprandial hyperinsulinemia. Interestingly, the beneficial effect of the pulse protein pattern on protein accretion still persisted several days after the end of the diet.[45] The pulse protein diet also restored a significant anabolic response of skeletal muscle protein synthesis to feeding without affecting protein breakdown in old rats.[46] These studies suggest that the use of a pulse protein pattern increases body protein retention, in particular in skeletal muscle. This concept represents a more attractive and safe approach than simply increased protein intake in the elderly population.

ANABOLIC RESPONSE TO PHYSICAL EXERCISE IN THE ELDERLY

Data from muscles in elderly men who have trained as swimmers, runners, or strength-trainers continuously for 12 to 17 years[47] suggest that long-term regular strength training in senescence can maintain the function and morphology of human skeletal muscles. Further study of both young and elderly strength-trained men will help establish whether strength training started in early adulthood results in further changes in skeletal muscle contractile properties.[48]

Many studies (for review see[49]) demonstrated that elderly people could significantly improve muscle strength and performance after a short period of high-intensity resistance training. These observations indicate that the capacity of muscle to adapt to resistance physical activity is preserved in old age even after a short period of training.[50] In addition, an interesting study[51] reported that the protein synthetic machinery adapts rapidly to increased contractile activity even in frail elders.

The anabolic effect of resistance exercise occurs via enhanced muscle protein synthesis. Yarasheski and colleagues[52] determined the rate of vastus lateralis muscle protein synthesis by using the in vivo incorporation of intravenously infused ^{13}C-leucine into mixed muscle protein in both young and elderly men before and at the end of 2 weeks of resistance exercise training. Although the muscle fractional synthesis rate was lower in the elderly before training, it increased to reach a comparable rate irrespective of the age of the subjects after 2 weeks of exercise. In contrast to these results, Welle and colleagues[53] found no improvement in myofibrillar protein synthesis rate in either young or old men who completed 12 weeks of resistance training. The discrepancy of these observations could be explained by the different experimental designs used in these studies. The training stimulus may not have been powerful enough to affect protein turnover in the investigation by Welle and colleagues.[53] In addition, the timing of the measurements relative to the last bout of exercise was also different in these investigations. Finally, the protein fraction (ie, myofibrillar fraction) used by Welle was different from that used by Yarasheski (ie, mixed muscle proteins). Other measurements of synthesis rate of individual muscle proteins showed that a 2-week weight-lifting program increased myosin heavy chain (MHC) synthesis rate in 23- to 32-year-old and 78- to 84-year-old subjects.[54] However, in this work the protein synthesis rate of actin was increased after exercise only in the younger group, showing that the anabolic effect of resistance exercise in elderly subjects is protein-dependent. Another work including young, middle-aged, and old people[55] demonstrated that age-related lowering of the transcript levels of MHC IIa and IIx is not reversed by 3 months of resistance exercise training, whereas exercise resulted in a higher synthesis rate of MHC in association with an increase in MHC I isoform transcript levels.[56] Other results[57] showed that the stimulation of MHC synthesis rate by resistance exercise is mediated by more efficient translation of mRNA. Furthermore, the effect of 16 weeks of endurance exercise on MHC isoform protein composition and mRNA abundance was tested in a recent study.[58] The regulation of MHC isoform transcripts remained robust in older muscle after endurance exercise, but this did not result in corresponding changes in MHC protein expression.

Few data are currently available concerning the rate of muscle protein breakdown after exercise in elderly subjects. Forty-five minutes of eccentric exercise produced a similar increase in whole-body protein breakdown irrespective of the age of the volunteers.[59] However, myofibrillar proteolysis, based on 3-methylhistidine–creatinine measurements, did not increase until 10 days postexercise in the young group but remained high through the same period in the older men. Interestingly, a recent study[60] determined the influence of age and resistance exercise on human skeletal muscle proteolysis by using a microdialysis approach. A higher interstitial 3-methylhistidine concentration was detected in the aged subjects. This suggested an increased proteolysis of contractile proteins in the rested and failed states. By contrast, interstitial 3-methylhistidine was not different from preexercise at any time point within 24 hours after exercise in both the young and elderly subjects.

Ageing muscle still responds to resistance or endurance training. Therefore, as shown by convincing data, exercise is beneficial to improve skeletal muscle strength and physical activity in elderly.

COMBINATION OF NUTRITIONAL AND TRAINING STRATEGIES

Most of the studies failed to show any beneficial effect of nutritional supplementations on muscle anabolic properties in exercising elderly subjects. For example, Welle and Thornton[61] reported that high-protein meals (0.6–2.4 g protein/kg/d) did not enhance the myofibrillar protein synthesis rate in vastus lateralis muscle after three sessions of resistance exercise in 62- to 75-year-old men and women. In frail very old people (87 years old), high-intensity resistance exercise training with or without concomitant multinutrient supplementation had the same efficiency on muscle weakness reversibility.[62] Of note, reports showed that ingestion of oral preexercise or postexercise amino acid supplements can improve net muscle protein balance in young volunteers.[63,64] The response to amino acid intake with concomitant exercise is dependent on the composition and amount, and the pattern and timing, of ingestion in relation to the performance of exercise.[65] The response of net muscle protein synthesis to consumption of an essential amino acid–carbohydrate supplement solution immediately before resistance exercise is greater than when the solution is consumed after exercise, primarily because of an increase in muscle protein synthesis as a result of increased delivery of amino acids to the leg.[66] Whether amino acid and carbohydrate intake immediately before or after resistance exercise can enhance the anabolic effect of training in older individuals as shown in the younger group remains to be determined.

HORMONAL IMPLICATIONS

Aging is associated with changes in several anabolic hormones, including insulin; the GH axis; the male sex hormones; and other steroid factors, such as dehydroepiandrosterone. Muscle fibers, like all cells, are regulated by these mediators. Only four hormones (insulin, GH, IGF-I, and testosterone) are covered here because reduced levels of these factors are likely to be the most important endocrine changes contributing to sarcopenia.[67]

Insulin

Insulin action during aging is altered for glucose uptake and use essentially. Response of amino acid metabolism to insulin has rarely been studied in aged volunteers and the results depend on the procedures used in the reports. At the whole-body level, clamp study in euglycemic but euaminoacidemic conditions has shown a subtle dysregulation of proteolysis to insulin at the whole-body level.[68] This reduced inhibition of protein degradation by insulin in elderly healthy subjects was also reproduced after meal intake.[68] In addition, recent work from Volpi and colleagues[21] may suggest some degree of insulin resistance for protein synthesis in aged muscle because addition of glucose decreased efficiency of amino acids mixture to promote protein synthesis in this population.

GH and IGF

There is an aged-associated decline in circulating GH[69] and the related-reduced stimulation of the liver signaling pathways by GH leads to decreased circulating levels of IGF-I in the elderly.[70] In addition, there is a decrease in IGF-I mRNA in older muscle that suggests a reduced local production of this growth factor.[71,72] IGF-I has several anabolic effects in muscle, including increased protein synthesis, enhancement of myoblast proliferation and differentiation, and neutrophic effects that enhance reinnervation of muscle fibers (for review see[73]). Additionally, low IGF-I levels were associated in healthy and frail older women with poor knee extensor muscle strength and slow walking speed.[74,75]

In humans, administration of recombinant GH to healthy older adults raises IGF-I levels and is reported to result in gains in total lean mass, muscle mass, and strength.[76–78] However, with GH, there is also the concern that the increase in lean mass is not accompanied by an increase in strength,[79] so it is not clear whether GH actually increases muscle protein or whether much of the lean body mass gain is in the visceral compartment. A recent study by Lange and colleagues[80] reported that GH administration during 12 weeks had no effect on isokinetic quadriceps muscle strength, cross-sectional area, or fiber size, but induced an increase in MHC two times isoform. In addition, IGF-I mRNA abundance was not increased in skeletal biopsy samples taken 10 hours after a subcutaneous injection of GH in men and women over 60 years of age.[81] These data do not support the hypothesis that increased IGF-I mRNA in skeletal muscle is required for the anabolic affect of GH in the elderly. In this study, there was also no effect of GH on levels of mRNA encoding the most abundant myofibrillar proteins, actin and MHC.[81] To the best of our knowledge, there are only two studies focusing on mixed muscle protein turnover during GH replacement in the healthy elderly and these experimentations reported discordant observations. Muscle protein synthesis was stimulated by 50% in one study[82] and not at all in the other.[78] However, the dose and duration of GH therapy differed.

Because the administration of GH can lead to undesirable side affects, such as carpal tunnel syndrome, interesting trials aimed at reestablishing GH secretory profiles by using GH releasing hormone (GHRH) treatment in elderly people.[83,84] GHRH injection for 4 months induced a significant increase in nocturnal GH levels, which was accompanied by increased serum concentrations of IGF-I.[83] In addition, lean body mass and nitrogen balance were improved in treated subjects compared with the placebo-controlled group. Another 6-week trial[84] demonstrated an increase in muscle strength and endurance, despite no change in lean body mass. In both cases, no significant side effects occurred after GHRH administration. More work is required with GHRH to assess the potential beneficial effect of such a treatment on muscle mass and function.

To avoid GH side effects, researchers have also explored the effects of IGF-I replacement. In mice, local overexpression of IGF-I in muscle prevents the age-related decline in muscle mass and strength.[85] IGF-I was also evaluated in humans at three different dosages and compared with GH.[82] Whole-body and mixed muscle protein synthesis were significantly increased by using high doses of IGF-I for 1 month.[82] Recently, Boonen and colleagues[86] noticed that improvement of muscle protein metabolism during IGF-I treatment was accompanied by elevated grip strength in frail elderly women. Again, these long-term studies revealed that IGF-I treatment had numerous negative side effects including headaches, lethargy, joint pain, and bloatedness.[87]

Whereas GH replacement has been shown to increase lean body mass and reduce body fat in GH-deficient adults, the benefits of GH, or IGF-I replacement therapy, in the healthy elderly are inconclusive and not without deleterious side effects. Myofibrillar protein synthesis and MHC synthesis rates are positively correlated to IGF-I levels,[88] but the short- and long-term effects of these hormones on individual muscle protein synthesis in the elderly have not been yet reported. GHRH administration may be a good solution with the aim to restore the GH–IGF-I axis anabolic properties in aged persons.

Testosterone

In men, the serum concentration of free testosterone declines by about 40% between the ages of 25 and 75 years.[89] In addition, circulating level of testosterone is correlated to muscle strength and MHC synthesis rate in elderly healthy subjects.[90,91] When elderly men were given replacement doses, which increased serum testosterone to a level comparable with that of young men, a significant gain in lean body mass and muscle strength was noted after 3 months.[92] Bilateral hand grip strength was also improved in 65-year-old hypogonadic men receiving, in double-blind, placebo-controlled study, 200 mg testosterone biweekly for 1 year.[93] Snyder and colleagues[94] randomized 108 hypogonadic men over 65 years of age to wear either a testosterone patch increasing the serum testosterone concentration to the physiologic range, or a placebo patch in a double-blind study for 36 months. These authors concluded that testosterone treatment increased lean body mass, principally in the trunk, but did not change the strength of knee extension and flexion, as measured by dynamometer.[94] The lack of an effect of testosterone on knee strength does not support the conventional knowledge about the properties of testosterone.[95] One possible explanation for this discrepancy is that the increase in serum testosterone concentration during treatment was not sufficiently great in this study. In addition, the muscle test used may not be the optimal test to detect appreciable changes in muscle strength. In previous works, muscle strength was assessed by hand grip, whereas Snyder and colleagues[94] evaluated the strength of knee extension and flexion. Ferrando and colleagues[96] recently demonstrated that older hypogonadic men receiving testosterone injection to maintain serum level that is mid-normal for healthy young men increased lean body mass and leg and arm strength after 6 months. In this study, lean body mass accretion resulted from an increase in muscle protein net balance because of a decrease in muscle protein breakdown. Only one other report has described the effect of hormone replacement on muscle protein turnover in elderly testosterone-deficient men.[97] These authors administered testosterone to six elderly men for 4 weeks, and found that mixed muscle protein synthesis was nearly double and several indices of leg strength increased. In addition, testosterone administration increased intramuscular mRNA concentrations of IGF-I and decreased mRNA for IGF-I binding proteins.[97] In another work, testosterone replacement also enhanced expression of IGF-I protein and androgen receptor within muscles of elderly hypogonadic patients.[96] These results were contradicted by Brill and colleagues,[98] who showed that normalization of testosterone level for 1 month by a transdermal patch had no effect on androgen receptor and myostatin gene expression in healthy older men with low serum testosterone level. Clinically speaking, this treatment improved 30-m walk and stair climb times in elderly subjects.[98]

Even though women express the androgen receptor, the importance of testosterone in maintaining their muscle mass and function is unclear. The fact that muscle mass and strength correlate with the total and free testosterone levels among 43- to 73-year-old women suggests that women produce enough testosterone to have anabolic effect.[99] Noticeably, restoration of youthful testosterone levels in postmenopausal women by administration of dehydroepiandrosterone, a precursor of testosterone, did not significantly improve muscle mass and strength.[100]

Taken together these results demonstrate that physiologic testosterone replacement in elderly men with low testosterone levels produces increases in muscle mass and strength. However, whether testosterone treatment can induce clinically meaningful changes in muscle function, reduce falls and fractures, or improve quality of life in older men is still unknown.[95] In addition, the potential side effects of these treatments include liver damage, prostate events, testicular atrophy, and dyslipidemia. The long-term safety of testosterone supplementation of older men, particularly with respect to the risk of cardiovascular disease and prostate cancer, remains to be established.

THERAPEUTIC CONSIDERATIONS

The possibility of any therapeutic approach to limit or prevent sarcopenia has been recently emphasized by studies linked to strategies aimed at limiting consequences of heart failure[101] or hypertension.[102,103] Therefore, when hypersensitive elderly subjects (mean age 78 years) are treated with angiotensin-converting enzyme inhibitor, a remarkable prevention of strength and walking speed decline has been noticed compared with other antihypertensive agents.[104] This is the first evidence of a pharmacologic approach being able to prevent age-related weakness. Many questions arise from this work, which represents an elegant invitation to apply important knowledge from the myocardic to the skeletal muscle.

SARCOPENIC OBESITY

The two greatest epidemiologic trends of our times are the obesity epidemic and the aging of the population.[105] The impact of obesity on mortality has decreased over time. This observation is consistent with the increased life expectancy among the obese population and the emergence of a new population segment, the obese elderly. Because aging and obesity are two conditions that represent an important part of health care spending, an increasingly obese elderly population will undoubtedly represent a growing financial problem in health care systems in economically developed countries.

A strong increase in obesity and overweight among elderly people (defined as a person $\geq$65 years of age) is reported in both sexes, all ages, all races, and all educational levels, both smokers and nonsmokers.[106–109] In this context, the prevalence of obesity among subjects aged 60 to 69 years was about 40% in the United States in the period of 1999 to 2000, 30% in those aged 70 to 79 years, and 20% in those aged 80 years and older.[110,111] In the United Kingdom, nearly 30% of people aged 55 to 65 years, 25% in those aged 65 to 75 years, and 20% in those aged 75 years or older are obese.[112] In France, the ObEpi study has reported that 16% of old people were obese in 2006 (ie, significantly more than in the general population). In French people aged 60 to 69 years, the prevalence of obesity was 18%, 17% in those aged 70 to 74 years, 16% in those aged 75 to 79 years, and 11% in those aged 80 years and older. In addition, the prevalence of overweight among elderly was about 40%.[113]

Definition of Sarcopenic Obesity

Sarcopenia displays major functional and metabolic consequences. This results in loss of muscle strength and contributes to the eventual inability of the elderly individual to carry out exercise or even tasks of daily living.[114,115] Sarcopenia contributes to the reduced ability to withstand physical activity in old age. Furthermore, decrease in muscle function can lead to a decrease in physical activity, thereby leading to osteoporosis, obesity, and impaired glucose tolerance.[116,117]

The depletion of muscle mass with age does not result in weight loss, suggesting that a corresponding accumulation of body fat occurs; hence, fat mass increases from 18% to 36% in elderly men.[118] Aging is also associated with a redistribution of body fat. With aging, there is a greater relative increase in intraabdominal, intrahepatic, and intramuscular fat than subcutaneous fat.[119] The size of intraabdominal depots is greater in old than in young adults at any given body mass index value. Changes in body fat distribution are associated with an increase in waist circumference in the elderly: about 0.7 cm per year between 40 and 70 years with no difference across age-strata (ie, even the oldest continued to have progressive increases in waist circumference).[120] In addition, abdominal fat accumulation is strongly associated with risk of metabolic disorders.[121,122]

Obesity in the elderly acts synergistically with sarcopenia to maximize disability. Sarcopenic obesity in old age is more strongly associated with disability than either sarcopenia or obesity per se.[123,124] Older people are particularly susceptible to the adverse effects of excess body weight because it can exacerbate the age-related decline in physical function (ie, the decrease in muscle mass and strength that occur with aging).

Metabolic Mediators of Sarcopenic Obesity

Inflammation

Aging is associated with increased levels of circulating inflammatory components in blood including elevated concentrations of cytokines and inflammatory proteins.[125–127] This chronic low-grade inflammation is associated with a variety of pathologic phenomena that affect the elderly, including sarcopenia, osteoporosis, atherosclerosis, reduced immune function, and insulin resistance.[128] Additionally, recent developments have demolished the concept that fat (ie, adipose cells) is metabolically inert. It is now well recognized that adipocytes actively participate in metabolic regulation, releasing fatty acids but also a wide range of protein factors and signals termed "adipokines" in an endocrine fashion. The secretome of adipocytes now numbers in excess of 100 different molecular entities. A number of adipokines, including adiponectin, leptin, TNF-α, IL-1β, IL-6, IL-8, IL-10, and monocyte chemoattractant protein-1 (MCP1) are linked to the inflammatory response. Hence, the white adipose tissue is considered as the main site of inflammation in obesity.[129] Obesity is therefore characterized by a state of inflammation that is closely associated with cardiovascular risks, insulin resistance, and metabolic syndrome. The basis for this view is that the circulating level of several cytokines (TNF-α, stNFR1, IL-6, and IL-18) and acute-phase proteins (C-reactive protein) associated with inflammation is increased in the obese.[130–133] In addition, weight loss in obese patients induced significant decreases in adipokine levels in both adipose tissue and serum.[134,135] Furthermore, adipocytes and macrophages colocalize in adipose tissue in obesity.[136] The arrival of macrophage in adipose tissue is likely to lead to a considerable amplification of the inflammatory state in white fat, and TNF-α plays a pivotal role in this infiltration. A key chemokine, MCP1, which is important in relation to attracting macrophages into a tissue, is released by adipocytes and expression and secretion of MCP1 is strongly upregulated by TNF-α.[137,138] In addition, it is well-known that macrophages secrete a variety of cytokines including TNF-α, IL-1β, and IL-6.

Increasing fat mass promotes production of TNF-α, IL-6, and other adipokines that further promote insulin resistance and potentially a direct catabolic effect on muscle (ie, enhancement of protein degradation and decrease in protein synthesis).

Lipotoxicity

An attractive new theory was advanced describing the accumulation of intratissue fat, particularly in muscle or liver, as responsible for the development of metabolic abnormalities in these tissues, in particular a decrease in insulin sensitivity and increased inflammatory state. For example, increased infiltration of lipids inside skeletal muscle leads to accumulation of lipid derivatives including long-chain acyl-CoAs, diacylglycerol, and ceramides, likely responsible for inhibition of intracellular biochemical pathway related to insulin action (ie, insulin signal transduction).[139–141] Moreover, the metabolic activity of the liver and pancreas is also impaired by an excess of intratissular fatty acids and this accumulation is involved in the development of type 2 diabetes mellitus.[142,143]

Recent studies have revealed that aging is accompanied by a change in the capacity to use and store dietary lipids. A significant ectopic lipid accumulation appears over time in humans as in animals, particularly in skeletal muscle. Very recently, the authors evaluated the effects of lipid infiltration on the loss of muscle anabolic ability with age. In this study, the authors observed a reduced plasticity of abdominal fat in old rats fed a high-fat diet (ie, obesigenic diet). A reduction in the size of adipocytes was noticed in old obese rats, which could be explained by the presence of numerous fibrous areas. The lesser expansion capacity of adipose tissue in older animals was associated with a very sharp increase in intramuscular lipid derivatives, such as triglycerides, diacyl glycerols, and ceramides. The appearance and development of insulin resistance associated with lipid overnutrition occurred earlier and took a greater extent in aged obese rats compared with younger obese rats. Interestingly, the rate of muscle protein synthesis was also reduced in obese aged rats compared with the young group.[144] This study also revealed the molecular link between accumulation of intramuscular lipid derivatives, such as ceramides, and reduced muscle protein synthesis. The alpha subunit of the eIF2 translational factor was hyperphosphorylated in older obese animals. Hyperphosphorylation of eIF2α leads to inhibition of protein synthesis. Therefore, the reduction in protein synthesis rate that was observed in older obese animals is likely related to an increased phosphorylation state of eIF2α itself induced by accumulation of lipid metabolites inside muscle cells.

Taken together, these new data clearly show that the capacity to adapt to lipid is blunted by age. These results also indicate that protein anabolism is nutritionally regulated not only by protein intake, but also by food lipids. This control is a cellular and molecular control because some lipid metabolites, such as ceramides, are able specifically to inhibit the rate of protein synthesis in skeletal muscle by modulating a key intermediate of protein translation, eIF2α. Thus, during aging, impaired expansion capacity of adipose tissue associated with ectopic fat accumulation, especially in muscle, has a dominant role in protein anabolism and may explain the acceleration of muscle protein loss during sarcopenic obesity.

Therefore, during aging, the physiologic loss of muscle mass (ie, sarcopenia) may occur as the primary event. This loss is a major contributor to decreased physical activity and energy expenditure and contributes to fat gain. This increased fat mass may in turn reinforce, through proinflammatory processes and lipotoxicity, muscle loss and abnormal muscle metabolism and function. A vicious cycle is created that leads to more gain in fat and more loss of muscle, until a threshold is crossed at which functional consequences, such as disability and illnesses, occur.

SUMMARY

Sarcopenia, like many other geriatric phenomena, involves a number of underlying mechanisms including intrinsic changes in the muscle and central nervous system and humoral and lifestyle factors. Muscle intrinsic changes include a decrease in the proportion in type II fibers, a reduction in mitochondrial and myofibrillar protein synthesis rates, and mitochondrial damages. Loss of alpha motor units from the spinal cord and alteration in hormone and cytokine production also affect muscle mass and function in the elderly. In addition, inadequate protein intake and physical inactivity are described to accelerate sarcopenia. However, the interactions between intrinsic and environmental factors associated with sarcopenia are not currently established.

Previous data have demonstrated that nutritional means to counter sarcopenia certainly exist. These strategies may gather an improvement of quality and pattern of the daily protein intake rather than simply increasing the amount of proteins, which should be cautiously used in an aged population with a potentially reduced kidney function. Moreover, inactivity also accelerates sarcopenia and resistance or endurance exercise reverses this phenomenon. Many studies have shown improvements in muscle function in response to strength training interventions in men and women of all ages, even the frail elderly. New data show that a combination of specific nutritional and physical activity programs might have a significant effect on muscle protein balance in young subjects. This strategy has to be tested in the long term in elderly people, especially those with increased body weight. Furthermore, the possibility of any therapeutic approach to limit sarcopenia has recently been emphasized in studies aiming initially to care for heart failure or hypertension. This pharmacologic approach might be combined to nutritional therapies.

REFERENCES

1. Janssen I, Shepard DS, Katzmarzyk PT, et al. The healthcare costs of sarcopenia in the United States. J Am Geriatr Soc 2004;52:80–5.
2. Walrand S, Boirie Y. Optimizing protein intake in aging. Curr Opin Clin Nutr Metab Care 2005;8:89–94.
3. Zadik Z, Chalew SA, McCarter RJ Jr, et al. The influence of age on the 24-hour integrated concentration of growth hormone in normal individuals. J Clin Endocrinol Metab 1985;60:513–6.
4. Rudman D, Feller A, Nagraj H, et al. Effects of human growth hormone in men over 60 years old. N Engl J Med 1990;323:1–6.
5. Papadakis MA, Grady D, Black D, et al. Growth hormone replacement in healthy older men improves body composition but not functional ability. Ann Intern Med 1996;124:708–16.
6. Nass R, Thorner MO. Impact of the GH–cortisol ratio on the age-dependent changes in body composition. Growth Horm IGF Res 2002;12:147–61.
7. Guillet C, Prod'homme M, Balage M, et al. Impaired anabolic response of muscle protein synthesis is associated with S6K1 dysregulation in elderly humans. FASEB J 2004;18:1586–7.
8. Fong Y, Moldawer LL, Marano M, et al. Cachectin/TNF or IL-1 alpha induces cachexia with redistribution of body proteins. Am J Physiol 1989;256(3 Pt 2): R659–65.
9. Lang CH, Frost RA, Nairn AC, et al. TNF-alpha impairs heart and skeletal muscle protein synthesis by altering translation initiation. Am J Physiol Endocrinol Metab 2002;282(2):E336–47.
10. Garcia-Martinez C, Agell N, Llovera M, et al. Tumour necrosis factor-alpha increases the ubiquitinization of rat skeletal muscle proteins. FEBS Lett 1993; 323(3):211–4.
11. Zoico E, Roubenoff R. The role of cytokines in regulating protein metabolism and muscle function. Nutr Rev 2002;60(2):39–51.
12. Biolo G, Declan Fleming RY, Wolfe RR. Physiologic hyperinsulinemia stimulates protein synthesis and enhances transport of selected amino acids in human skeletal muscle. J Clin Invest 1995;95(2):811–9.
13. Guillet C, Zangarelli A, Gachon P, et al. Whole body protein breakdown is less inhibited by insulin, but still responsive to amino acid, in nondiabetic elderly subjects. J Clin Endocrinol Metab 2004;89(12):6017–24.
14. Carbo N, Ribas V, Busquets S, et al. Short-term effects of leptin on skeletal muscle protein metabolism in the rat. J Nutr Biochem 2000;11(9):431–5.
15. Walrand S, Vasson MP, Lesourd B. The role of nutrition in immunity of the aged. In: Perdigon G, Fuller R, editors. Gut flora, nutrition and immunity. Oxford (United Kingdom): Blackwell; 2003. p. 237–69.
16. Short KR, Nair KS. The effect of age on protein metabolism. Curr Opin Clin Nutr Metab Care 2000;3:39–44.
17. Volpi E, Ferrando AA, Yeckel CW, et al. Exogenous amino acids stimulate net muscle protein synthesis in the elderly. J Clin Invest 1998;101:2000–7.
18. Volpi E, Mittendorfer B, Wolf SE, et al. Oral amino acids stimulate muscle protein anabolism in the elderly despite higher first-pass splanchnic extraction. Am J Physiol 1999;277:E513–20.

19. Boirie Y, Gachon P, Beaufrere B. Splanchnic and whole-body leucine kinetics in young and elderly men. Am J Clin Nutr 1997;65:489–95.
20. Volpi E, Kobayashi H, Sheffield-Moore M, et al. Essential amino acids are primarily responsible for the amino acid stimulation of muscle protein anabolism in healthy elderly adults. Am J Clin Nutr 2003;78:250–8.
21. Volpi E, Mittendorfer B, Rasmussen BB, et al. The response of muscle protein anabolism to combined hyperaminoacidemia and glucose-induced hyperinsulinemia is impaired in the elderly. J Clin Endocrinol Metab 2000;85:4481–90.
22. Mosoni L, Valluy MC, Serrurier B, et al. Altered response of protein synthesis to nutritional state and endurance training in old rats. Am J Physiol 1995;268: E328–35.
23. Rand WM, Pellett PL, Young VR. Meta-analysis of nitrogen balance studies for estimating protein requirements in healthy adults. Am J Clin Nutr 2003;77: 109–27.
24. Campbell WW, Crim MC, Dallal GE, et al. Increased protein requirements in elderly people: new data and retrospective reassessments. Am J Clin Nutr 1994;60:501–9.
25. Campbell WW, Evans WJ. Protein requirements of elderly people. Eur J Clin Nutr 1996;50(Suppl 1):S180–3 [discussion: S183–5].
26. Millward DJ, Fereday A, Gibson N, et al. Aging, protein requirements, and protein turnover. Am J Clin Nutr 1997;66:774–86.
27. Millward DJ. Optimal intakes of protein in the human diet. Proc Nutr Soc 1999; 58:403–13.
28. Gaillard C, Alix E, Boirie Y, et al. Are elderly hospitalized patients getting enough protein? J Am Geriatr Soc 2008;56:1045–9.
29. Pannemans DL, Halliday D, Westerterp KR. Whole-body protein turnover in elderly men and women: responses to two protein intakes. Am J Clin Nutr 1995;61:33–8.
30. Walrand S, Short K, Bigelow M, et al. Effect of a high protein diet on insulin sensitivity, leucine kinetics, and renal function in healthy elderly humans. Am J Physiol Endocrinol Metab 2008.
31. Castaneda C, Dolnikowski GG, Dallal GE, et al. Protein turnover and energy metabolism of elderly women fed a low-protein diet. Am J Clin Nutr 1995;62:40–8.
32. Castaneda C, Charnley JM, Evans WJ, et al. Elderly women accommodate to a low-protein diet with losses of body cell mass, muscle function, and immune response. Am J Clin Nutr 1995;62:30–9.
33. Houston DK, Nicklas BJ, Ding J, et al. Dietary protein intake is associated with lean mass change in older, community-dwelling adults: the Health, Aging, and Body Composition (Health ABC) Study. Am J Clin Nutr 2008;87:150–5.
34. Pannemans DL, Wagenmakers AJ, Westerterp KR, et al. Effect of protein source and quantity on protein metabolism in elderly women. Am J Clin Nutr 1998;68: 1228–35.
35. Boirie Y, Dangin M, Gachon P, et al. Slow and fast dietary proteins differently modulate postprandial protein accretion. Proc Natl Acad Sci U S A 1997;94: 14930–5.
36. Dangin M, Guillet C, Garcia-Rodenas C, et al. The rate of protein digestion affects protein gain differently during aging in humans. J Physiol 2003;549: 635–44.
37. Paddon-Jones D, Sheffield-Moore M, Katsanos CS, et al. Differential stimulation of muscle protein synthesis in elderly humans following isocaloric ingestion of amino acids or whey protein. Exp Gerontol 2006;41:215–9.

38. Paddon-Jones D, Short KR, Campbell WW, et al. Role of dietary protein in the sarcopenia of aging. Am J Clin Nutr 2008;87(Suppl):1562S–6S.
39. Dardevet D, Sornet C, Balage M, et al. Stimulation of in vitro rat muscle protein synthesis by leucine decreases with age. J Nutr 2000;130:2630–5.
40. Dardevet D, Sornet C, Bayle G, et al. Postprandial stimulation of muscle protein synthesis in old rats can be restored by a leucine-supplemented meal. J Nutr 2002;132:95–100.
41. Guillet C, Zangarelli A, Mishellany A, et al. Mitochondrial and sarcoplasmic proteins, but not myosin heavy chain, are sensitive to leucine supplementation in old rat skeletal muscle. Exp Gerontol 2004;39:745–51.
42. Anthony JC, Anthony TG, Kimball SR, et al. Signaling pathways involved in translational control of protein synthesis in skeletal muscle by leucine. J Nutr 2001;131:856S–60S.
43. Rieu I, Sornet C, Bayle G, et al. Leucine-supplemented meal feeding for ten days beneficially affects postprandial muscle protein synthesis in old rats. J Nutr 2003;133:1198–205.
44. Arnal MA, Mosoni L, Boirie Y, et al. Protein pulse feeding improves protein retention in elderly women. Am J Clin Nutr 1999;69:1202–8.
45. Arnal MA, Mosoni L, Boirie Y, et al. Protein turnover modifications induced by the protein feeding pattern still persist after the end of the diets. Am J Physiol Endocrinol Metab 2000;278:E902–9.
46. Arnal MA, Mosoni L, Dardevet D, et al. Pulse protein feeding pattern restores stimulation of muscle protein synthesis during the feeding period in old rats. J Nutr 2002;132:1002–8.
47. Klitgaard H, Mantoni M, Schiaffino S, et al. Function, morphology and protein expression of ageing skeletal muscle: a cross-sectional study of elderly men with different training backgrounds. Acta Physiol Scand 1990;140:41–54.
48. Evans WJ, Campbell WW. Sarcopenia and age-related changes in body composition and functional capacity. J Nutr 1993;123:465–8.
49. Hurley BF, Hagberg JM. Optimizing health in older persons: aerobic or strength training? Exerc Sport Sci Rev 1998;26:61–89.
50. Roubenoff R. Sarcopenia: a major modifiable cause of frailty in the elderly. J Nutr Health Aging 2000;4:140–2.
51. Schulte JN, Yarasheski KE. Effects of resistance training on the rate of muscle protein synthesis in frail elderly people. Int J Sport Nutr Exerc Metab 2001; 11(Suppl):S111–8.
52. Yarasheski KE, Zachwieja JJ, Bier DM. Acute effects of resistance exercise on muscle protein synthesis rate in young and elderly men and women. Am J Physiol 1993;265:E210–4.
53. Welle S, Thornton C, Statt M. Myofibrillar protein synthesis in young and old human subjects after three months of resistance training. Am J Physiol 1995; 268:E422–7.
54. Hasten DL, Pak-Loduca J, Obert KA, et al. Resistance exercise acutely increases MHC and mixed muscle protein synthesis rates in 78–84 and 23–32 yr olds. Am J Physiol Endocrinol Metab 2000;278:E620–6.
55. Balagopal P, Schimke JC, Ades P, et al. Age effect on transcript levels and synthesis rate of muscle MHC and response to resistance exercise. Am J Physiol Endocrinol Metab 2001;280:E203–8.
56. Williamson DL, Godard MP, Porter DA, et al. Progressive resistance training reduces myosin heavy chain coexpression in single muscle fibers from older men. J Appl Physiol 2000;88:627–33.

57. Welle S, Bhatt K, Thornton CA. Stimulation of myofibrillar synthesis by exercise is mediated by more efficient translation of mRNA. J Appl Physiol 1999;86:1220-5.
58. Short KR, Vittone JL, Bigelow ML, et al. Changes in myosin heavy chain mRNA and protein expression in human skeletal muscle with age and endurance exercise training. J Appl Physiol 2005;99:95-102.
59. Fielding RA, Meredith CN, O'Reilly KP, et al. Enhanced protein breakdown after eccentric exercise in young and older men. J Appl Physiol 1991;71:674-9.
60. Trappe T, Williams R, Carrithers J, et al. Influence of age and resistance exercise on human skeletal muscle proteolysis: a microdialysis approach. J Physiol 2004; 554:803-13.
61. Welle S, Thornton CA. High-protein meals do not enhance myofibrillar synthesis after resistance exercise in 62- to 75-yr-old men and women. Am J Physiol 1998; 274:E677-83.
62. Fiatarone MA, O'Neill EF, Ryan ND, et al. Exercise training and nutritional supplementation for physical frailty in very elderly people. N Engl J Med 1994;330:1769-75.
63. Tipton KD, Ferrando AA, Phillips SM, et al. Postexercise net protein synthesis in human muscle from orally administered amino acids. Am J Physiol 1999;276: E628-34.
64. Tipton KD, Borsheim E, Wolf SE, et al. Acute response of net muscle protein balance reflects 24 H balance following exercise and amino acid ingestion. Am J Physiol Endocrinol Metab 2002;11:11.
65. Wolfe RR. Regulation of muscle protein by amino acids. J Nutr 2002;132: 3219S-24S.
66. Tipton KD, Rasmussen BB, Miller SL, et al. Timing of amino acid-carbohydrate ingestion alters anabolic response of muscle to resistance exercise. Am J Physiol Endocrinol Metab 2001;281:E197-206.
67. Welle S. Cellular and molecular basis of age-related sarcopenia. Can J Appl Physiol 2002;27:19-41.
68. Boirie Y, Gachon P, Cordat N, et al. Differential insulin sensitivities of glucose, amino acid, and albumin metabolism in elderly men and women. J Clin Endocrinol Metab 2001;86:638-44.
69. Rosen CJ. Growth hormone and aging. Endocrine 2000;12:197-201.
70. Janssen JA, Lamberts SW. Is the measurement of free IGF-I more indicative than that of total IGF-I in the evaluation of the biological activity of the GH/ IGF-I axis? J Endocrinol Invest 1999;22:313-5.
71. Goldspink G. Cellular and molecular aspects of muscle growth, adaptation and ageing. Gerodontology 1998;15:35-43.
72. Hameed M, Harridge SD, Goldspink G. Sarcopenia and hypertrophy: a role for insulin-like growth factor-1 in aged muscle? Exerc Sport Sci Rev 2002;30:15-9.
73. Rooyackers OE, Nair KS. Hormonal regulation of human muscle protein metabolism. Annu Rev Nutr 1997;17:457-85.
74. Cappola AR, Bandeen-Roche K, Wand GS, et al. Association of IGF-I levels with muscle strength and mobility in older women. J Clin Endocrinol Metab 2001;86: 4139-46.
75. Kostka T, Arsac LM, Patricot MC, et al. Leg extensor power and dehydroepiandrosterone sulfate, insulin-like growth factor-I and testosterone in healthy active elderly people. Eur J Appl Physiol 2000;82:83-90.
76. Hennessey JV, Chromiak JA, DellaVentura S, et al. Growth hormone administration and exercise effects on muscle fiber type and diameter in moderately frail older people. J Am Geriatr Soc 2001;49:852-8.

77. Rudman D, Feller AG, Nagraj HS, et al. Effects of human growth hormone in men over 60 years old. N Engl J Med 1990;323:1–6.

78. Welle S, Thornton C, Statt M, et al. Growth hormone increases muscle mass and strength but does not rejuvenate myofibrillar protein synthesis in healthy subjects over 60 years old. J Clin Endocrinol Metab 1996;81:3239–43.

79. Yarasheski KE, Zachwieja JJ, Campbell JA, et al. Effect of growth hormone and resistance exercise on muscle growth and strength in older men. Am J Physiol 1995;268:E268–76.

80. Lange KH, Andersen JL, Beyer N, et al. GH administration changes myosin heavy chain isoforms in skeletal muscle but does not augment muscle strength or hypertrophy, either alone or combined with resistance exercise training in healthy elderly men. J Clin Endocrinol Metab 2002;87:513–23.

81. Welle S, Thornton C. Insulin-like growth factor-I, actin, and myosin heavy chain messenger RNAs in skeletal muscle after an injection of growth hormone in subjects over 60 years old. J Endocrinol 1997;155:93–7.

82. Butterfield GE, Thompson J, Rennie MJ, et al. Effect of rhGH and rhIGF-I treatment on protein utilization in elderly women. Am J Physiol 1997;272:E94–9.

83. Khorram O, Laughlin GA, Yen SS. Endocrine and metabolic effects of long-term administration of [Nle27]growth hormone-releasing hormone-(1-29)-NH2 in age-advanced men and women. J Clin Endocrinol Metab 1997;82:1472–9.

84. Vittone J, Blackman MR, Busby-Whitehead J, et al. Effects of single nightly injections of growth hormone-releasing hormone (GHRH 1-29) in healthy elderly men. Metabolism 1997;46:89–96.

85. Barton-Davis ER, Shoturma DI, Musaro A, et al. Viral mediated expression of insulin-like growth factor I blocks the aging-related loss of skeletal muscle function. Proc Natl Acad Sci U S A 1998;95:15603–7.

86. Boonen S, Rosen C, Bouillon R, et al. Musculoskeletal effects of the recombinant human IGF-I/IGF binding protein-3 complex in osteoporotic patients with proximal femoral fracture: a double-blind, placebo-controlled pilot study. J Clin Endocrinol Metab 2002;87:1593–9.

87. Thompson JL, Butterfield GE, Marcus R, et al. The effects of recombinant human insulin-like growth factor-I and growth hormone on body composition in elderly women. J Clin Endocrinol Metab 1995;80:1845–52.

88. Waters DL, Baumgartner RN, Garry PJ. Sarcopenia: current perspectives. J Nutr Health Aging 2000;4:133–9.

89. Vermeulen A, Kaufman JM, Giagulli VA. Influence of some biological indexes on sex hormone-binding globulin and androgen levels in aging or obese males. J Clin Endocrinol Metab 1996;81:1821–6.

90. Balagopal P, Rooyackers OE, Adey DB, et al. Effects of aging on in vivo synthesis of skeletal muscle myosin heavy-chain and sarcoplasmic protein in humans. Am J Physiol 1997;273:E790–800.

91. van den Beld AW, de Jong FH, Grobbee DE, et al. Measures of bioavailable serum testosterone and estradiol and their relationships with muscle strength, bone density, and body composition in elderly men. J Clin Endocrinol Metab 2000;85:3276–82.

92. Tenover JS. Effects of testosterone supplementation in the aging male. J Clin Endocrinol Metab 1992;75:1092–8.

93. Sih R, Morley JE, Kaiser FE, et al. Testosterone replacement in older hypogonadal men: a 12-month randomized controlled trial. J Clin Endocrinol Metab 1997;82:1661–7.

94. Snyder PJ, Peachey H, Hannoush P, et al. Effect of testosterone treatment on body composition and muscle strength in men over 65 years of age. J Clin Endocrinol Metab 1999;84:2647–53.
95. Bross R, Storer T, Bhasin S. Aging and Muscle Loss. Trends Endocrinol Metab 1999;10:194–8.
96. Ferrando AA, Sheffield-Moore M, Yeckel CW, et al. Testosterone administration to older men improves muscle function: molecular and physiological mechanisms. Am J Physiol Endocrinol Metab 2002;282:E601–7.
97. Urban RJ, Bodenburg YH, Gilkison C, et al. Testosterone administration to elderly men increases skeletal muscle strength and protein synthesis. Am J Physiol 1995;269:E820–6.
98. Brill KT, Weltman AL, Gentili A, et al. Single and Combined Effects of Growth Hormone and Testosterone Administration on Measures of Body Composition, Physical Performance, Mood, Sexual Function, Bone Turnover, and Muscle Gene Expression in Healthy Older Men. J Clin Endocrinol Metab 2002;87: 5649–57.
99. Hakkinen K, Pakarinen A. Muscle strength and serum testosterone, cortisol and SHBG concentrations in middle-aged and elderly men and women. Acta Physiol Scand 1993;148:199–207.
100. Morales AJ, Haubrich RH, Hwang JY, et al. The effect of six months treatment with a 100 mg daily dose of dehydroepiandrosterone (DHEA) on circulating sex steroids, body composition and muscle strength in age-advanced men and women. Clin Endocrinol (Oxf) 1998;49:421–32.
101. Parmley WW. Evolution of angiotensin-converting enzyme inhibition in hypertension, heart failure, and vascular protection. Am J Med 1998;105:27S–31S.
102. Schaufelberger M, Andersson G, Eriksson BO, et al. Skeletal muscle changes in patients with chronic heart failure before and after treatment with enalapril. Eur Heart J 1996;17:1678–85.
103. Vescovo G, Dalla Libera L, Serafini F, et al. Improved exercise tolerance after losartan and enalapril in heart failure: correlation with changes in skeletal muscle myosin heavy chain composition. Circulation 1998;98:1742–9.
104. Onder G, Penninx BW, Balkrishnan R, et al. Relation between use of angiotensin-converting enzyme inhibitors and muscle strength and physical function in older women: an observational study. Lancet 2002;359:926–30.
105. Roubenoff R. Sarcopenic obesity: the confluence of two epidemics. Obes Res 2004;12(6):887–8.
106. Flegal KM, Carroll MD, Ogden CL, et al. Prevalence and trends in obesity among US adults, 1999–2000. JAMA 2002;288(14):1723–7.
107. Gutierrez-Fisac JL, Lopez E, Banegas JR, et al. Prevalence of overweight and obesity in elderly people in Spain. Obes Res 2004;12(4):710–5.
108. Mokdad AH, Bowman BA, Ford ES, et al. The continuing epidemics of obesity and diabetes in the United States. JAMA 2001;286(10):1195–200.
109. Mokdad AH, Ford ES, Bowman BA, et al. Prevalence of obesity, diabetes, and obesity-related health risk factors. JAMA 2003;289(1):76–9.
110. Zamboni M, Mazzali G, Zoico E, et al. Health consequences of obesity in the elderly: a review of four unresolved questions. Int J Obes (Lond) 2005;29(9): 1011–29.
111. Flegal KM, Wei R, Ogden C. Weight-for-stature compared with body mass index-for-age growth charts for the United States from the Centers for Disease. Control and Prevention. Am J Clin Nutr 2002;75(4):761–6.

112. Seidell JC. Prevalence and time trends of obesity in Europe. J Endocrinol Invest 2002;25(10):816–22.
113. Enquête ObEpi 2006: réalisée par TNS Healthcare Sofres auprès de 23.747 adultes (15 ans et plus) et financée par la firme Roche (Institut Roche de l'Obésité), 4ème enquête après celles de 1997, 2000 et 2003.
114. Rantanen T, Guralnik JM, Sakari-Rantala R, et al. Disability, physical activity, and muscle strength in older women: the Women's Health and Aging Study. Arch Phys Med Rehabil 1999;80(2):130–5.
115. Short KR, Nair KS. Muscle protein metabolism and the sarcopenia of aging. Int J Sport Nutr Exerc Metab 2001;11:S119–27.
116. Dutta C, Hadley EC. The significance of sarcopenia in old age. J Gerontol 1996; 50A:1–4.
117. Evans WJ. What is sarcopenia? J Gerontol A Biol Sci Med Sci 1995;50 Spec No: 5–8.
118. Walrand S, Boirie Y. Muscle protein and amino acid metabolism with respect to age-related sarcopenia. In: Cynober LA, editor. Amino acid metabolism and therapy in health and nutritional disease. Boca Raton: CRC Press; 2004. p. 389–404.
119. Beaufrere B, Morio B. Fat and protein redistribution with aging: metabolic considerations. Eur J Clin Nutr 2000;54:S48–53.
120. Noppa H. Body weight change in relation to incidence of ischemic heart disease and change in risk factors for ischemic heart disease. Am J Epidemiol 1980; 111(6):693–704.
121. Farin HM, Abbasi F, Reaven GM. Body mass index and waist circumference both contribute to differences in insulin-mediated glucose disposal in nondiabetic adults. Am J Clin Nutr 2006;83(1):47–51.
122. Racette SB, Evans EM, Weiss EP, et al. Abdominal adiposity is a stronger predictor of insulin resistance than fitness among 50–95 year olds. Diabetes Care 2006;29(3):673–8.
123. Baumgartner RN, Wayne SJ, Waters DL, et al. Sarcopenic obesity predicts instrumental activities of daily living disability in the elderly. Obes Res 2004; 12(12):1995–2004.
124. Rolland Y, Lauwers-Cances V, Cristini C, et al. Difficulties with physical function associated with obesity, sarcopenia, and sarcopenic-obesity in community-dwelling elderly women: the EPIDOS (EPIDemiologie de l'OSteoporose) Study. Am J Clin Nutr 2009;89(6):1895–900.
125. Bruunsgaard H, Pedersen M, Pedersen BK. Aging and proinflammatory cytokines. Curr Opin Hematol 2001;8(3):131–6.
126. Walrand S, Moreau K, Caldefie F, et al. Specific and nonspecific immune responses to fasting and refeeding differ in healthy young adult and elderly persons. Am J Clin Nutr 2001;74(5):670–8.
127. Walrand S, Vasson M-P, Lesourd B. The role of nutrition in immunity of the aged. In: Perdigon G, Fuller R, editors. Gut flora, nutrition and immunity. Oxford: Blackwells; 2003. p. 237–69.
128. Kennedy RL, Chokkalingham K, Srinivasan R. Obesity in the elderly: who should we be treating, and why, and how? Curr Opin Clin Nutr Metab Care 2004;7(1): 3–9.
129. Trayhurn P. Endocrine and signalling role of adipose tissue: new perspectives on fat. Acta Physiol Scand 2005;184(4):285–93.
130. Bullo M, Garcia-Lorda P, Megias I, et al. Systemic inflammation, adipose tissue tumor necrosis factor, and leptin expression. Obes Res 2003;11(4):525–31.

131. Engstrom G, Hedblad B, Stavenow L, et al. Inflammation-sensitive plasma proteins are associated with future weight gain. Diabetes 2003;52(8):2097–101.
132. Festa A, D'Agostino R Jr, Williams K, et al. The relation of body fat mass and distribution to markers of chronic inflammation. Int J Obes Relat Metab Disord 2001;25(10):1407–15.
133. Yudkin JS, Stehouwer CD, Emeis JJ, et al. C-reactive protein in healthy subjects: associations with obesity, insulin resistance, and endothelial dysfunction: a potential role for cytokines originating from adipose tissue? Arterioscler Thromb Vasc Biol 1999;19(4):972–8.
134. Bastard JP, Jardel C, Bruckert E, et al. Elevated levels of interleukin 6 are reduced in serum and subcutaneous adipose tissue of obese women after weight loss. J Clin Endocrinol Metab 2000;85(9):3338–42.
135. Esposito K, Pontillo A, Di Palo C, et al. Effect of weight loss and lifestyle changes on vascular inflammatory markers in obese women: a randomized trial. JAMA 2003;289(14):1799–804.
136. Wellen KE, Hotamisligil GS. Inflammation, stress, and diabetes. J Clin Invest 2005;115(5):1111–9.
137. Wang B, Jenkins JR, Trayhurn P. Expression and secretion of inflammation-related adipokines by human adipocytes differentiated in culture: integrated response to TNF-alpha. Am J Physiol Endocrinol Metab 2005;288(4):E731–40.
138. Adams JM II, Pratipanawatr T, Berria R, et al. Ceramide content is increased in skeletal muscle from obese insulin-resistant humans. Diabetes 2004;53(1): 25–31.
139. Shulman GI. Cellular mechanisms of insulin resistance. J Clin Invest 2000; 106(2):171–6.
140. Kim JK, Fillmore JJ, Chen Y, et al. Tissue-specific overexpression of lipoprotein lipase causes tissue-specific insulin resistance. Proc Natl Acad Sci U S A 2001; 98(13):7522–7.
141. Yki-Järvinen H. Fat in the liver and insulin resistance. Ann Med 2005;37(5): 347–56.
142. Boden G, Shulman GI. Free fatty acids in obesity and type 2 diabetes: defining their role in the development of insulin resistance and beta-cell dysfunction. Eur J Clin Invest 2002;32(Suppl 3):14–23.
143. Tardif N, Salles J, Guillet C, et al. The increased sensitivity to the deleterious effects of high fat diet in old rats is related to an increase in muscle ceramide levels during aging. Amsterdam: European congress of obesity; 2009.
144. Tardif N, Salles J, Guillet C, et al. High fat diet decreases muscle protein synthesis in aged rats: Involvement of intramuscular ceramide accumulation. First International Congress of Translational Research in Human Nutrition. Clermont-Ferrand; 2010.

Consequences of Sarcopenia

Marjolein Visser, PhD[a,b,*], Laura A. Schaap, PhD[b]

KEYWORDS

• Muscle mass • Muscle strength • Disability
• Mortality • Falls • Aged

This article discusses the consequences of sarcopenia in older persons. The focus is on three specific consequences: (1) functional status, (2) falls, and (3) mortality. The described relationship between sarcopenia and these outcomes is based on the results of epidemiologic studies in large cohorts of older men and women.

The original definition of sarcopenia refers to the age-related loss of muscle mass. However, it is important to realize that as yet very limited data have been published on repeated measures of muscle mass in older persons to establish that the age-related change is muscle mass and to subsequently relate this change to negative health outcomes. Therefore, this overview is mainly based on both cross-sectional and longitudinal, epidemiologic studies using a single assessment of muscle mass. In these studies, the health outcomes of older persons with a lower muscle mass have been compared with those of older persons with a higher muscle mass. In other studies the term "sarcopenia" was used to define older persons with a low muscle mass. These sarcopenic persons were then contrasted with older persons with a normal muscle mass to investigate potential differences in various health outcomes.

In the scientific literature the term "sarcopenia" has also been used in a much broader sense, for example to indicate the age-related loss of muscle strength or the presence of poor muscle strength in older persons. In this article, the term "dynapenia" is used to describe this process. Sarcopenia and dynapenia are distinct processes with different pathophysiology. Although the two processes may occur simultaneously in some individuals, they do not necessarily overlap.[1] The use of these

The authors have nothing to disclose.
[a] Faculty of Earth and Life Sciences, Department of Health Sciences, VU University Amsterdam, De Boelelaan 1085, 1081 HV Amsterdam, The Netherlands
[b] EMGO+ Institute, Department of Epidemiology and Biostatistics, VU University Medical Center, Van der Boechorststraat 7, 1081 BT Amsterdam, The Netherlands
* Corresponding author. Faculty of Earth and Life Sciences, Department of Health Sciences, VU University Amsterdam, De Boelelaan 1085, 1081 HV Amsterdam, The Netherlands.
E-mail address: marjolein.visser@falw.vu.nl

Clin Geriatr Med 27 (2011) 387–399
doi:10.1016/j.cger.2011.03.006
0749-0690/11/$ – see front matter © 2011 Elsevier Inc. All rights reserved.
geriatric.theclinics.com

two different terms allows a clear distinction between the consequences of low muscle mass and those of low muscle strength.

SARCOPENIA AND FUNCTIONAL STATUS

Several cross-sectional, observational studies have related sarcopenia to measures of functional status, such as mobility performance, self-reported functional limitations, and disability.[2-6] In the New Mexico Elder Health Survey, appendicular skeletal muscle mass (ASMM) was estimated using a prediction equation that included weight, height, hip circumference, grip strength, and gender. Sarcopenia was defined as having a ratio of ASMM/height^2 less than 7.26 for men and less than 5.45 for women. Sarcopenia was significantly associated with a threefold to fourfold increased risk of self-reported physical disability in both men and women.[2] Sarcopenia measured as skeletal muscle mass index (SMI = the ratio of skeletal muscle mass by bioelectrical impedance divided by total body mass) in men and women enrolled in the National Health and Nutrition Examination Survey (NHANES) study was associated with an increased need of assistance with personal care or handling routine daily chores.[3] These findings were confirmed in an Italian study among 167 community-dwelling women aged 67 to 78 years. After adjustment for age and several chronic diseases, women with an SMI less than or equal to two times the standard deviation (SD) of a young reference group (120 premenopausal healthy women) had a 3.8 times increased risk of having functional limitations compared with women with normal SMI values.[4] In the Health, Aging, and Body Composition (Health ABC) study, older adults in the lowest skeletal muscle quintile (adjusted for height and fat mass) were 80% to 90% more likely to have mobility impairment than older persons in the highest quintile.[5] In another study using data from the Health ABC study, smaller mid-thigh muscle cross-sectional area, assessed by CT scans, was significantly associated with poorer performance on a 6-m walk test and a repeated chair-stands test in older men and women.[6]

In contrast to the previously mentioned studies, other epidemiologic studies failed to observe an association between sarcopenia and functional status. These studies include older[7,8] and more recent[9-11] cross-sectional studies and several prospective studies.[12,13] In the Framingham Heart Study, total body and lower-extremity muscle mass by dual-energy x-ray absorptiometry (DXA) were not associated with disability using a nine-item questionnaire among 753 men and women aged 72 to 95 years.[7] In a large, community-based cohort of 1655 men and women aged 55 years and older, lean mass as estimated from bioelectrical impedance measurements was not associated with self-reported functional limitations after adjustment for age, fat mass, height, chronic disease, physical activity, and smoking.[8] After adjustment, higher lean mass was associated with faster, objectively assessed walking speed in men but not in women.

More recent cross-sectional studies confirm these findings. In 109 men and women aged 60 years and older, ASMM as assessed by DXA was not associated with performance test scores or self-reported functional limitations.[9] Using data from the EPIDOS study including women aged 75 years and older, the association between sarcopenia and limitations performing activities of daily living was investigated.[10] Women were classified as sarcopenic if their relative ASMM corrected for height was less than or equal to two SDs below the mean of a reference population from the Rosetta Study, which included healthy Americans aged 18 to 40 years.[14] Sarcopenia was not associated with having difficulty in performing daily activities, such as walking and climbing stairs.[10] Data from the InChianti Study indicated that sarcopenia of the calf muscle, assessed using CT, had little influence on walking speed, a powerful predictor of incident disability and frailty in older persons.[11]

Two prospective studies consistently reported a lack of association between low muscle mass and incident functional limitations or disability. In the Cardiovascular Health Study, fat-free mass as estimated from bioelectrical impedance measurements was not associated with 3-year incidence of self-reported disability based on 17 tasks among 1489 men and 1785 women aged 65 to 100 years.[12] Another prospective study reported that lower thigh muscle cross-sectional area was not associated with the incidence of mobility limitations during a 2.5-year follow-up among well-functioning men and women aged 70 to 79 years after adjustment for muscle strength and fat infiltration.[13]

To our knowledge, only one small study examined changes in body composition and their relationship with incidence of self-reported disability in older persons.[15] Ninety-seven women and 62 men aged 71.4 (SD 2.2) years and 71.6 (SD 2.2) years, respectively, underwent DXA determinations and reported their disability level at baseline and after 2 and 5.5 years of follow-up. After adjustment for gender and chronic diseases, persons who lost ASMM (cut-off at median change in muscle mass) had a 2.15-fold increased risk of having a worsening disability compared with persons who remained stable. For decline in leg skeletal muscle mass the increased risk was 2.53-fold.

Regarding the relationship between sarcopenia and functional status, it can be concluded that although early, cross-sectional studies reported significant associations, most recent studies and prospective studies found weak or no associations between sarcopenia and functional status. These studies do not, however, provide information on whether loss of skeletal muscle mass in old age is detrimental to functional status. Only one study suggested that loss of muscle mass may parallel a decline in self-reported disability level and more research is warranted to confirm these findings.[15]

DYNAPENIA AND FUNCTIONAL STATUS

Poor muscle strength is a well-known determinant of poor functional status based on observational studies.[13,16–19] A recent cross-sectional study using data from NHANES showed that leg strength was associated with impaired functional status. The association remained significant after adjustment for age, sex, alcohol intake, smoking status, chronic diseases, and physical activity level.[16] In a longitudinal study in which older men and women from the Health ABC study were followed for 2.5 years, low knee extensor strength was associated with a higher risk of mobility limitations. After adjustment for age, race, study site, body height, and total body fat mass, men and women in the lowest quartile of muscle strength were 2.64 (95% confidence interval [CI], 1.83–3.80) and 2.15 (95% CI, 1.61–2.87) times more likely to develop mobility limitations compared with those in the highest quartile of muscle strength. After additional adjustment for other potential confounders, including lifestyle and health factors, the association remained statistically significant.[13] Although this study also observed an association between mid-thigh muscle area and increased risk of mobility limitations, this risk was not independent of poor muscle strength. Other observational studies investigating both low muscle mass and poor muscle strength in relationship to functional status in older persons consistently showed a strong association between muscle strength and function, with no or much weaker associations between muscle mass and function.[17,18] Thus, at least in the wide range of study samples of community-dwelling older persons used in these studies, the function of the muscle seems more relevant in relationship to functional status in old age compared with muscle size.

The life history of muscle strength may also impact functional status in old age. A study of Rantanen and colleagues[20] showed that grip strength assessed in a large sample of healthy Japanese-American men aged 45 to 68 years was highly predictive of functional limitations and disability 25 years later when all participants were at least 70 years of age. These results suggest that high muscle strength throughout life may contribute to the prevention of disability later in life.

It can be concluded that dynapenia is strongly associated with functional status. Although initial studies reported the importance of muscle mass, new data are beginning to shift the paradigm toward muscle weakness as a major risk factor for mobility limitations and disability in old age.

SARCOPENIA AND FALLS

Sarcopenia is frequently mentioned as an important risk factor for falls in older persons. However, there are not many epidemiologic studies that specifically have addressed the association between skeletal muscle mass in old age and the risk of falls. The results of two studies are presented next, although in both studies the fall data were collected retrospectively; at the time of the muscle mass assessment the falls that occurred in the previous 12 months were reported. Among 883 elderly Hispanic and non-Hispanic white men and women with mean age 74 years living in New Mexico (the New Mexico Elder Health Survey) the association between sarcopenia and reported falls in the past year was studied.[2] ASMM was estimated using a prediction equation that included weight, height, hip circumference, grip strength, and gender. Sarcopenia was defined as having a ratio of ASMM/height^2 less than 7.26 for men and less than 5.45 for women. Twenty-two percent of the men and 31% of the women reported a fall in the past year. After adjustment for age, ethnicity, obesity, comorbidity, and alcohol intake, the odds ratio (OR) for falls was statistically significant in men at 2.58 (95% CI, 1.42–4.73) but not in women at 1.28 (95% CI, 0.60–2.67). The second study investigating the association between muscle mass and falls was conducted in 796 men aged 50 to 85 years of age who participated in the MINOS study. Relative appendicular muscle mass (RASM = ASMM by DXA divided by body height$^{2.3}$) was related to self-reported falls in the past 12 months.[21] Of the men, 25.4% reported a fall in the past year. After adjustment for age, body weight, serum free testosterone and vitamin D concentration, and chronic diseases, the OR per SD lower RASM was 1.31 (95% CI, 1.03–1.65). Men in the highest tertile of RASM (>7.31 kg/m$^{2.3}$) were less likely to report a fall in the previous year compared with those in the lowest quartile of RASM (<6.32 kg/m$^{2.3}$; OR 0.66 [95% CI, 0.44–0.99]).

In contrast to the extensive research focusing on the relationship between low muscle mass and functional status, only two studies have examined the relationship between low muscle mass and falls. In both studies muscle mass was assessed after the falls were experienced. It therefore cannot be excluded that muscle mass has been negatively affected by the experience of falls (eg, caused by an increased fear of falling and related decreased physical activity level) or by the potential consequences of the fall (injuries). Although both studies reported that low muscle mass was associated with more reported falls, reverse causation cannot be excluded from these studies and the results should be interpreted carefully. No prospective studies have investigated the relationship between loss of muscle mass and fall risk in older persons.

DYNAPENIA AND FALLS

Compared with the association between sarcopenia and fall risk, the association between dynapenia and fall risk has been studied more extensively. A meta-analysis was conducted based on 30 cohort studies that were published between January 1985 and March 2002, met the inclusion criteria, and investigated the relationship between baseline measurements of muscle strength and prospective data on fall occurrence.[22] At least 50% of the study sample had to be age 65 years or older. Of this selection, 13 independent studies were available for data extraction. Knee extension, ankle dorsiflexion, and chair stands were the most common measures used to assess lower-extremity weakness. The combined OR for the association between lower-extremity weakness and any fall based on six individual studies was 1.76 (95% CI, 51.31–2.37). The combined estimated OR for the association between lower-extremity weakness and recurrent falls was even higher (3.06 [95% CI, 1.86–5.04]) based on six different studies. For injurious falls, the meta-analysis showed an estimated OR of 1.52 (95% CI, 51.05–2.20) for the relationship with lower-extremity muscle weakness. However, this estimate was only based on two studies. Upper-extremity weakness was assessed by grip strength or manual muscle testing in most studies. The ORs for upper-extremity weakness were statistically significant but of a lower magnitude than the ORs for lower-extremity weakness. For example, for recurrent falls, the meta-analysis showed an estimated OR of 1.41 (1.25–1.59) for upper-extremity weakness.

Since the publication of this meta-analysis, new studies have been published examining the association between muscle strength and falls. Several studies developed a prediction model to predict future fall risk and identified poor muscle strength as an important predictor in the model. For example, during a follow-up period of 36 weeks, 33% of 311 community-dwelling persons aged 70 years and older reported 197 falls at 6-weekly telephone calls.[23] Poor grip strength (≤ 12 kg for women and ≤ 22 kg for men) assessed at baseline was a predictor of recurrent falls in the final risk model (OR 3.1 [95% CI, 1.5–6.6]), which also included previous falls, abnormal postural sway, and depressive symptoms. A second example is a Dutch study in which fall data were prospectively collected during a 3-year follow-up in 1365 community-dwelling men and women aged 65 years and older participating in the Longitudinal Aging Study Amsterdam.[24] The incidence of recurrent falls during follow-up was 24.9% in women and 24.4% in men. Men and women with a grip strength in the lowest 20th percentile (≤ 32 kg for women and ≤ 56 kg for men) were more likely to experience greater than or equal to two falls during a 6-month period compared with those with higher grip strength (OR 2.32; 95% CI, 1.71–3.13). Poor grip strength remained a statistically significant predictor of recurrent falling in a risk profile also including previous falling, dizziness, functional limitations, low body weight, high education, high alcohol consumption, fear of falling, and cats or dogs in the household. In this model, the OR of the association between poor grip strength and recurrent falls was 1.74 (95% CI, 1.19–2.54). A final example is the Women's Health and Aging Study, in which an algorithm was developed to predict any future fall among 1002 community-dwelling women aged 65 years old or older with disability.[25] The best performing algorithm included previous falls, and in selected subpopulations balance problems, walking speed, body mass index, and knee extensor strength. These three examples clearly show the ability of poor muscle strength to predict future fall risk in older men and women, supporting the important role of dynapenia in falls of older persons.

To our knowledge, no observational studies have investigated the association between change in muscle strength and future risk of falls. However, there is clear evidence from intervention studies that exercise decreases the risk of future falls in older men and women.[26] However, the specific contribution of increased muscle strength caused by the exercise intervention in preventing falls independent of other positive effects of the exercise intervention (eg, on balance, sway, or depressive symptoms) has not yet been established.

SARCOPENIA AND MORTALITY

Several epidemiologic studies used anthropometrically assessed muscle mass, usually a measure of mid-arm muscle circumference or mid-arm muscle area as calculated from mid-arm circumference and skinfold thickness, to investigate the association between low muscle mass and mortality. A study among 1396 men and women aged 70 years and older showed that after adjustment for baseline age, gender, marital status, smoking, self-rated health, ability to conduct activities of daily living, comorbidity, cognition performance, and presence of depression, low arm muscle area ($\leq$21.4 cm^2 for men and $\leq$21.6 cm^2 for women) was associated with 8-year mortality risk (hazard ratio [HR] 1.95; 95% CI, 1.25–2.00).[27] The relationship between arm muscle area (square centimeter) and mortality was also studied in 957 community-dwelling Japanese men and women aged 65 to 102 years.[28] During the 2-year follow-up 236 persons died. In multivariate analyses, adjusting for age, gender, functional status, comorbidity status, and triceps skinfold thickness as a measure of body fatness, low arm muscle area (<23.5 cm^2) was associated with a higher mortality risk (HR 2.03; 95% CI, 1.36–3.02) compared with high arm muscle area ($\geq$33.4 cm^2). Mortality risk was highest for those persons who had a low arm muscle and a low triceps skinfold thickness (HR 3.83; 95% CI, 1.97–7.47). Among 4107 British men aged 60 to 79 years low mid-arm muscle circumference was associated with increased risk of mortality during a 6-year follow-up.[29] Men in the highest quartile of mid-arm muscle circumference ($\geq$27.94 cm) were less likely to die (HR 0.71; 95% CI, 0.56–0.88) compared with men in the lowest quartile of muscle circumference (<24.91 cm) after adjustment for age, social class, physical activity, alcohol intake, and smoking. This association persisted after additional adjustment for lung function, serum albumin, weight loss, height loss, self-reported poor health, preexisting cancer, diabetes, and cardiovascular disease; the HR for men in the highest muscle circumference quartile was 0.73 (95% CI, 0.58–0.92). Finally, an association between arm muscle area and 24-year mortality was also observed among 452 men aged 65 years and older.[30] After adjustment for age, height, smoking, social class, physical activity, chronic disease, caloric intake, reported weight loss, percent body fat (from skinfolds), and grip strength, the HR per SD higher arm muscle area was 0.86 (95% CI, 0.76–0.98) in men. In the 348 women the HR was 0.94 (95% CI, 0.81–1.08) and not statistically significant. These large studies using upper arm muscle circumference (centimeter) or area (square centimeter) as a rather crude measure of muscle mass quite consistently suggest that low upper body muscle mass is associated with an increased risk of mortality in older men and women.

Other studies investigating the relationship between muscle mass and mortality have been using total body fat-free mass as an indicator of skeletal muscle mass. Similar to the studies using anthropometrically assessed muscle mass, these studies should be carefully interpreted because they did not directly measure muscle mass. Fat-free mass also includes other lean tissues including visceral lean mass. The results of these studies are less consistent compared with the studies using anthropometric muscle measurements. Lower levels of fat-free mass as estimated from potassium 40 counting were associated with an increased mortality risk among 787 men aged 60 years and older who were followed for 22 years.[31] In a large study among 57,053 Danish men and women 50 to 64 years old, low fat-free mass (estimated from bioelectrical impedance) divided by body height squared was associated with increased

6-year mortality risk independent of fat mass.[32] In contrast, in the Study of Osteoporotic Fractures quintiles of fat-free mass estimated from bioelectrical impedance measurements were not associated with mortality during an 8-year follow-up in 8029 women aged 65 years and older.[33] The HR of mortality was 1.16 (95% CI, 0.92–1.45) for women in the highest quintile of fat-free mass versus those in the lowest quintile of fat-free mass, after adjustment for age, smoking, self-reported health, grip strength, nonthiazide diuretic use, and femoral neck bone mineral density. When restricting the analyses to never-smokers only, the HR for low fat-free mass increased to 1.32 but was still not statistically significant. Similarly, quintiles of fat-free mass as assessed by underwater weighing or the sum of seven skinfolds were not associated with 12-year mortality (P for trend 0.91) among 2603 men and women aged 60 to 100 years after adjustment for age, gender, examination year, smoking status, abnormal exercise electrocardiogram responses, baseline health conditions, and cardiorespiratory fitness.[34] These findings are in line with those of Wannamethee and colleagues[29] who showed that quartiles of the fat-free mass index, as estimated from bioelectrical impedance measurements, were not associated with 6-year mortality in 4107 British men aged 60 to 79 years (P for trend 0.42).

More recently, large epidemiologic studies have used accurate body composition methodology to assess skeletal muscle mass in older men and women. CT has been used to assess regional muscle cross-sectional area, usually at the mid-thigh level. DXA has also been used to measure ASMM or skeletal muscle mass only of the legs. The studies investigating the association between accurately assessed muscle mass and mortality are reviewed in detail because they provide the strongest evidence on the relationship between muscle mass and mortality. Data from the Health, Aging and Body composition study among 2292 well-functioning older men and women aged 70 to 79 years living in the Memphis and Pittsburgh regions of the United States were used to study the association between muscle mass and mortality.[35] The mean follow-up was 4.9 years during which 286 persons (12.5%) died. Both leg skeletal muscle mass from DXA and mid-thigh muscle cross-sectional area from CT were used. Moreover, many potential confounders were considered including age; race; chronic diseases; smoking status; level of physical activity; mid-thigh fat area by CT or total body fat mass by DXA; height; and markers of inflammation, including interleukin-6, C-reactive protein, and tumor necrosis factor-α. In men and women, leg skeletal muscle mass expressed per SD (1.8 kg) was not associated with mortality. Mid-thigh muscle area was associated with mortality risk in men. Per SD (28.1 cm^2) lower muscle area the HR was 1.26 (95% CI, 1.02–1.55). However, in women no association was observed (HR 0.94; 95% CI, 0.66–1.35). In a publication some years later, data from 934 Italian men and women aged 65 years or older, participants of the InChianti study who were followed for 6 years, were used to study the association between muscle mass and mortality.[11] Muscle cross-sectional area (square centimeter) of the calf was measured using peripheral quantitative CT. Although unadjusted analyses showed a lower mortality risk per SD higher muscle area (HR 0.75; 95% CI, 0.66–0.86), this association disappeared after considering potential confounders. After adjusting for height, weight, age, gender, study site, education, cognitive status, depressive symptoms, physical activity, and chronic disease, the HR increased to 0.86 (95% CI, 0.68–1.08) and was no longer statistically significant. Muscle density (milligram per cubic centimeter) of the calf muscle was also not related to mortality risk. These findings have been recently confirmed by a French study among 715 men aged 50 to 85 years.[36] During the 10 years of follow-up 137 men (19.2%) died. Baseline ASMM was not associated with mortality after adjustment for potential confounding. Men in the lowest quartile of muscle mass were not more likely to die during the follow-up period (OR 1.08; 99% CI, 0.54–2.15) compared with those in the highest quartile. These three studies consistently show that having a low skeletal muscle mass, based on a single assessment of muscle mass, is not a determinant of mortality in older men and women.

To our knowledge only two prospective studies have examined the change in muscle mass over time in older persons and its relationship with mortality risk. In the Framingham Heart Study, 2-year change in total body fat-free mass was estimated using repeated bioelectrical impedance measurements in 398 men and women aged 72 to 92 years at baseline.[37] The fat-free mass index was calculated by dividing fat-free mass (kilogram) by body height (meter) squared and served as a proxy of muscle mass. Greater loss of fat-free mass was associated with increased mortality in the subsequent 2 years, during which 55 persons (13.8%) died. After adjustment for gender, body mass index, smoking, being bedridden, C-reactive protein level, arthritis, cardiovascular disease, diabetes, and levels of different cytokines, the HR per unit decline in fat-free mass index was 1.9 (95% CI ,1.3–2.6). Researchers from the MINOS study recently investigated the change in accurately assessed skeletal muscle mass by DXA in relationship to mortality.[36] These unique analyses were conducted among 715 older men who were followed for 7.5 years with DXA measurements conducted every 18 months. The rate of loss in total body lean soft tissue per year was not different between those who died during the 10-year mortality follow-up and those who survived ($P = .24$). However, the rate of loss of ASMM per year was faster in those who died (–315.5 [SD 364.3] g/y) compared with those who survived (–182.5 [SD 190.9] g/y; $P<.0001$). When expressed as the relative rate of loss per year the difference was statistically significant (–1.43% vs –0.78%; $P<.0001$). After adjustment for potential confounders, including age, body mass index, height, smoking, educational level, occupational physical activity, frailty index, prevalent ischemic heart disease, diabetes, aortic calcification score, 17β-estradiol, and serum 25–hydroxycholecalciferol, one SD decrease in ASMM was associated with a higher mortality risk (HR 1.61; 99% CI, 1.28–2.01). Even after additional adjustment for weight loss in the multivariate models, men in the lowest tertile of ASMM loss (losing more than 264 g/y) had a higher mortality risk (HR 2.27; 99% CI, 1.19–4.33) compared with men in the highest tertile of loss (losing <114 g/y). This final analysis suggests that accelerated muscle mass loss, independent of weight loss, might be a strong determinant of mortality in older persons.

Although observational studies that have used rather crude assessments of skeletal muscle mass based on anthropometry suggest that low muscle mass might be associated with increased mortality risk, studies using a single measurement of accurately assessed muscle mass consistently show that low muscle mass is not a determinant of mortality in older men and women. However, there is some recent evidence that accelerated loss of skeletal muscle mass, irrespective of weight loss, might be a risk factor for early mortality in older persons.

DYNAPENIA AND MORTALITY

With regard to the association between measures of muscle strength and mortality risk in older persons, the research findings have been far more consistent compared with the association between measures of muscle mass and mortality. Many studies have been published showing an inverse association between grip strength, frequently used as a proxy of overall body strength in old age, and mortality. For example, in men aged 65 years and older, poor grip strength was a strong determinant of 25-year mortality risk independent of physical activity and muscle mass as assessed by 24-hour creatinine excretion.[38] Among 919 moderately to severely disabled women aged 65 to 101 years, those in the lowest tertile of grip strength were twice more likely to die from cardiovascular disease (RR 2.17; 95% CI, 1.26–3.73) compared with those in the highest tertile after adjusting for age, race, body height, and weight.[39] Similar results were observed for all-cause mortality and further adjustments for multiple diseases, physical inactivity, smoking, interleukin-6, C-reactive protein, serum albumin, unintentional weight loss, and depressive symptoms did not materially attenuate the risk estimates, suggesting that grip strength may influence mortality through mechanisms other than those leading from disease to muscle impairment. More recent data from 2292 well-functioning older men and women aged 70 to 79 years who were followed for a mean of 4.9 years showed an increased mortality risk per SD (10.7 kg) lower grip strength in men (HR 1.36; 95% CI, 1.13–1.64) and in women (HR 1.84; 95% CI, 1.28–2.65).[35] After adjustment for age, race, comorbidities, smoking status, level of physical activity, body composition as assessed by DXA, height, and several markers of inflammation these estimates were only slightly attenuated: HR 1.36 (95% CI, 1.10–1.60) for men and 1.67 (95% CI, 1.08–2.58) for women. An association between lower grip strength and 24-year mortality was observed among 452 men aged 65 years and older.[30] After adjustment for age, height, smoking, social class, physical activity, chronic disease, caloric intake, reported weight loss, arm muscle area, and percent body fat from skinfolds, the mortality HR per SD in grip strength was 0.81 (95% CI, 0.70–0.94). In women, however, the association was not statistically significant (HR 1.10; 95% CI, 0.86–1.40). Lower grip strength in men was also associated with cancer mortality, cardiovascular mortality, and respiratory mortality.

Other studies have extended these findings with other measures of muscle strength. In 960 older persons with a mean age of 87 years a higher extremity muscle strength, a composite strength measure of nine muscle groups ranging from pinch strength to ankle dorsiflexion, was associated with a lower risk of mortality during a follow-up of 2.2 years (HR 0.56; 95% CI, 0.38–0.83) after adjustment for age, gender, education, and body mass index.[40] In the Health ABC study, a 48-Nm lower isokinetic quadriceps strength was associated with an increased risk of mortality in men and women (HR 1.51 [95% CI, 1.28–1.79] and HR 1.65 [95% CI, 1.19–2.30], respectively).[35] After full adjustment these HRs changed to 1.45 (95% CI, 1.21–1.74) in men and 1.47 (95% CI, 1.02–2.14) in women and remained statistically significant. Additional adjustment for mid-thigh muscle cross-sectional area by CT or leg lean mass by CT only slightly attenuated these estimates. Finally, an association between muscle power and mortality has been reported. Arm-cranking power was stronger associated with 40-year mortality than isometric arm strength (a composite measure of eight arm strength measures and grip strength) among 993 middle-aged men.[41] The relative risk for mortality per 100 kg/m/min of arm-cranking power was 0.987 (95% CI, 0.978–0.996) after adjustment for age, body mass index, height, physical activity, and creatinine excretion and remained statistically significant even after additional adjustment for isometric arm strength.

Similar to the studies on the relationship between loss of muscle mass and mortality, only a few studies have investigated the association of age-related change in muscle strength over time with mortality risk. In men aged 60 years and older, higher grip strength was more strongly associated with 40-year mortality risk than the rate of grip strength loss over a period of 25 years. This association persisted when muscle mass, as estimated by 24-hour creatinine excretion, and physical activity were considered.[38] In a single proportional hazards model, the rate of change in muscle strength (kilogram per year) per year was a stronger determinant of 40-year mortality

(HR 0.854; 95% CI, 0.809–0.901) compared with the actual muscle strength (HR 0.955; 95% CI, 0.935–0.976), although the relationship of both muscle parameters with mortality was statistically significant.[41] In a study among 837 persons with a mean age of 81 years at baseline, 36% experienced a decline in muscle strength over 2.2 years as estimated by ordinary least squares regression with a term for time from baseline in years.[42] During follow-up, 9.7% of the study sample died. For each unit increase in muscle strength over time a lower mortality risk was observed, even after adjustment for baseline muscle strength, age, gender, education, and body mass index (HR 0.898; 95% CI, 0.809–0.996).

With regard to the association between dynapenia and mortality risk in old age, it can be concluded that the literature provides clear evidence that poor isometric muscle strength, poor isokinetic muscle strength, and poor muscle power are determinants of mortality in older men and women. The literature also showed that indicators of low muscle mass did not explain this association and only attenuated the risk estimates to a small extent. The few prospective studies conducted in older persons seem to suggest that both the actual level of muscle strength and the age-related loss of muscle strength play a role in mortality risk in old age.

SUMMARY

Based on the results of these epidemiologic studies conducted in large samples of older men and women it can be concluded that poor muscle functioning, as indicated by poor muscle strength or poor muscle power, increases the risk of functional decline, falls, and mortality. The impact of poor muscle functioning was stronger and more consistent throughout the different studies compared with the impact of low muscle mass. Furthermore, there is evidence that the relationship between poor muscle strength and these three different outcomes is not, or very limited, influenced by the size of the muscle. Based on the limited number of studies focusing on the age-related loss of muscle mass in relationship with the three different outcomes, there is some evidence suggesting that loss of muscle mass might increase the risk of functional decline and mortality. Further prospective studies are needed to investigate the relationship between accurately assessed loss of muscle mass and loss of muscle strength using repeated measurements with functional status, falls, and mortality in older persons.

REFERENCES

1. Clark BC, Manini TM. Sarcopenia ≠ dynapenia. J Gerontol A Biol Sci Med Sci 2008;63:829–34.
2. Baumgartner RN, Koehler KM, Gallagher D, et al. Epidemiology of sarcopenia among the elderly in New Mexico. Am J Epidemiol 1998;147(8):755–63.
3. Janssen I, Heymsfield SB, Ross R. Low relative skeletal muscle mass (sarcopenia) in older persons is associated with functional impairment and physical disability. J Am Geriatr Soc 2002;50(5):889–96.
4. Zoico E, Di Francesco V, Guralnik JM, et al. Physical disability and muscular strength in relation to obesity and different body composition indexes in a sample of healthy elderly women. Int J Obes Relat Metab Disord 2004; 28(2):234–41.
5. Newman AB, Kupelian V, Visser M, et al. Sarcopenia: alternative definitions and associations with lower extremity function. J Am Geriatr Soc 2003;51(11): 1602–9.

6. Visser M, Kritchevsky SB, Goodpaster BH, et al. Leg muscle mass and composition in relation to lower extremity performance in man and women aged 70–79: the Health, Aging and Body Composition study. J Am Geriatr Soc 2002; 50(5):897–904.

7. Visser M, Harris TB, Langlois J, et al. Body fat and skeletal muscle mass in relation to physical disability in very old men and women of the Framingham Heart Study. J Gerontol A Biol Sci Med Sci 1998;53:M214–21.

8. Sternfeld B, Ngo L, Satariano WA, et al. Associations of body composition with physical performance and self-reported functional limitation in elderly men and women. Am J Epidemiol 2002;156(2):110–21.

9. Jankowski CM, Gozansky WS, Van Pelt RE, et al. Relative contributions of adiposity and muscularity to physical function in community-dwelling older adults. Obesity (Silver Spring) 2008;16:1039–44.

10. Rolland Y, Lauwers-Cances V, Cristini C, et al. Difficulties with physical function associated with obesity, sarcopenia, and sarcopenic-obesity in community-dwelling elderly women: the EPIDOS (EPIDemiologie de l'OSteoporose) Study. Am J Clin Nutr 2009;89:1895–900.

11. Cesari M, Pahor M, Lauretani F, et al. Skeletal muscle and mortality results from the InCHIANTI Study. J Gerontol A Biol Sci Med Sci 2009;64(3):377–84.

12. Visser M, Langlois J, Guralnik JM, et al. High body fatness, but not low fat-free mass, predicts disability in older men and women: the Cardiovascular Health Study. Am J Clin Nutr 1998;68(3):584–90.

13. Visser M, Goodpaster BH, Kritchevsky SB, et al. Muscle mass, muscle strength, and muscle fat infiltration as predictors of incident mobility limitations in well-functioning older persons. J Gerontol A Biol Sci Med Sci 2005; 60:324–33.

14. Gallagher D, Visser M, de Meersman RE, et al. Appendicular skeletal muscle mass: effects of age, gender, and ethnicity. J Appl Physiol 1997;83(1): 229–39.

15. Fantin F, Di Francesco V, Fontana G, et al. Longitudinal body composition changes in old men and women: interrelationships with worsening disability. J Gerontol A Biol Sci Med Sci 2007;62(12):1375–81.

16. Bouchard DR, Janssen I. Dynapenic-obesity and physical function in older adults. J Gerontol A Biol Sci Med Sci 2010;65(1):71–7.

17. Visser M, Deeg DJ, Lips P, et al. Skeletal muscle mass and muscle strength in relation to lower-extremity performance in older men and women. J Am Geriatr Soc 2000;48:381–6.

18. Lauretani F, Russo CR, Bandinelli S, et al. Age-associated changes in skeletal muscles and their effect on mobility: an operational diagnosis of sarcopenia. J Appl Physiol 2003;95(5):1851–60.

19. Ferrucci L, Penninx BW, Volpato S, et al. Change in muscle strength explains accelerated decline of physical function in older women with high interleukin-6 serum levels. J Am Geriatr Soc 2002;50:1947–54.

20. Rantanen T, Guralnik JM, Foley D, et al. Midlife hand grip strength as a predictor of old age disability. JAMA 1999;281:558–60.

21. Szulc P, Beck TJ, Marchand F, et al. Low skeletal muscle mass is associated with poor structural parameters of bone and impaired balance in elderly men–The MINOS Study. J Bone Miner Res 2005;20:721–9.

22. Moreland JD, Richardson JA, Goldsmith CH, et al. Weakness and falls in older adults: a systematic review and meta-analysis. J Am Geriatr Soc 2004; 52:1121–9.

23. Stalenhoef PA, Diederiks JP, Knottnerus JA, et al. A risk model for the prediction of recurrent falls in community-dwelling elderly: a prospective cohort study. J Clin Epidemiol 2002;55:1088–94.

24. Pluijm SM, Smit JH, Tromp EA, et al. A risk profile for identifying community-dwelling elderly with a high risk of recurrent falling: results of a 3-year prospective study. Osteoporos Int 2006;17:417–25.

25. Lamb SE, McCabe C, Becker C, et al. The optimal sequence and selection of screening test items to predict fall risk in older disabled women: the Women's Health and Aging Study. J Gerontol A Biol Sci Med Sci 2008;63: 1082–8.

26. Gillespie LD, Robertson MC, Gillespie WJ, et al. Interventions for preventing falls in older people living in the community. Cochrane Database Syst Rev 2009;2: CD007146.

27. Miller MD, Crotty M, Giles LC, et al. Corrected arm muscle area: an independent predictor of long-term mortality in community-dwelling older adults? J Am Geriatr Soc 2002;50:1272–7.

28. Enoki H, Kuzuya M, Masuda Y, et al. Anthropometric measurements of mid-upper arm as a mortality predictor for community-dwelling Japanese elderly: the Nagoya Longitudinal Study of Frail Elderly (NLS-FE). Clin Nutr 2007;26: 597–604.

29. Wannamethee SG, Shaper AG, Lennon L, et al. Decreased muscle mass and increased central adiposity are independently related to mortality in older men. Am J Clin Nutr 2007;86:1339–46.

30. Gale CR, Martyn CN, Cooper C, et al. Grip strength, body composition, and mortality. Int J Epidemiol 2007;36:228–35.

31. Heitmann BL, Erikson H, Ellsinger BM, et al. Mortality associated with body fat, fat-free mass and body mass index among 60-year-old Swedish men: a 22-year follow-up. The study of men born in 1913. Int J Obes Relat Metab Disord 2000;24:33–7.

32. Bigaard J, Frederiksen K, Tjonneland A, et al. Body fat and fat-free mass and all-cause mortality. Obes Res 2004;12:1042–9.

33. Dolan CM, Kraemer H, Browner W, et al. Associations between body composition, anthropometry, and mortality in women aged 65 years and older. Am J Public Health 2007;97:913–8.

34. Sui X, LaMonte MJ, Laditka JN, et al. Cardiorespiratory fitness and adiposity as mortality predictors in older adults. JAMA 2007;298:2507–16.

35. Newman AB, Kupelian V, Visser M, et al. Strength, but not muscle mass, is associated with mortality in the health, aging and body composition study cohort. J Gerontol A Biol Sci Med Sci 2006;61:72–7.

36. Szulc P, Munoz F, Marchand F, et al. Rapid loss of appendicular skeletal muscle mass is associated with higher all-cause mortality in older men: the prospective MINOS study. Am J Clin Nutr 2010;91:1227–36.

37. Roubenoff R, Parise H, Payette HA, et al. Cytokines, insulin-like growth factor 1, sarcopenia, and mortality in very old community-dwelling men and women: the Framingham Heart Study. Am J Med 2003;115:429–35.

38. Metter EJ, Talbot LA, Schrager M, et al. Skeletal muscle strength as a predictor of all-cause mortality in healthy men. J Gerontol A Biol Sci Med Sci 2002;57: B359–65.

39. Rantanen T, Volpato S, Ferrucci L, et al. Handgrip strength and cause-specific and total mortality in older disabled women: exploring the mechanism. J Am Geriatr Soc 2003;51:636–41.

40. Buchman AS, Boyle PA, Wilson RS, et al. Pulmonary function, muscle strength and mortality in old age. Mech Ageing Dev 2008;129:625–31.
41. Metter EJ, Talbot LA, Schragger M, et al. Arm-cranking muscle power and arm isometric muscle strength are independent predictors of all-cause mortality in men. J Appl Physiol 2004;96:814–21.
42. Buchman AS, Wilson RS, Boyle PA, et al. Change in motor function and risk of mortality in older persons. J Am Geriatr Soc 2007;55:11–9.

Sarcopenia and Obesity

Debra L. Waters, PhD[a],*, Richard N. Baumgartner, PhD[b]

KEYWORDS

• Sarcopenia • Obesity • Sarcopenic obesity • Aging

It is now widely accepted that 4 body composition phenotypes exist in older adults: normal, sarcopenic, obese, and a combination of sarcopenic and obese. There is still no consensus, however, on the definitions and classifications of these phenotypes and their etiology and consequences continue to be debated. The lack of standard definitions, particularly for sarcopenia and sarcopenic obesity, creates challenges for determining their prevalence across different populations. It is recognized that the etiology of these phenotypes is multifactorial with complex covariate relationships. This review focuses on the current literature addressing the classification, prevalence, etiology, and correlates of sarcopenia, obesity, and the combination of sarcopenia and obesity referred to in this review as sarcopenic obesity.

DEFINING OBESITY, SARCOPENIA, AND SARCOPENIC OBESITY

Assessing skeletal muscle or fat mass in elders in clinical settings is challenging without the use of precise methods, such as dual energy x-ray absorptiometry (DXA), magnetic resonance spectroscopy, or axial CT scans. As a result, clinical assessments often rely on anthropometric methods that may be subject to substantial misclassification errors. The most widely used clinical measure for assessing obesity is body mass index (BMI).[1,2] BMI is calculated as weight (kg)/height squared (m²), with adult scores ranging from less than 18.5 (underweight) to greater than 40 (extreme obesity) (**Table 1**).

The BMI cut scores used to define obesity were derived from increases in all-cause mortality associated with a BMI above 30 kg/m². The loss of height and lean body mass and increasing fat mass during aging, however, uncouple the relationship between BMI and obesity, thereby attenuating associations with mortality.[2,3] The loss of height results in an overestimation of fatness, whereas a decrease in lean body mass under-estimates fatness. Because of this, it has been argued that BMI cut scores are not

[a] Department of Preventive and Social Medicine, Dunedin School of Medicine, University of Otago, PO Box 913, Dunedin 9054, New Zealand
[b] Department of Epidemiology and Population Health, University of Louisville, 485 East Gray Street, Louisville, KY 40202, USA
* Corresponding author.
E-mail address: debra.waters@otago.ac.nz

Clin Geriatr Med 27 (2011) 401–421
doi:10.1016/j.cger.2011.03.007
0749-0690/11/$ – see front matter © 2011 Elsevier Inc. All rights reserved.

Table 1 Body mass index classifications		
Classification	BMI (kg/m²)	Obesity Class
Underweight	<18.5	
Normal	18.5–24.9	
Overweight	25.0–29.9	I
Obesity	30.0–39.9	II
Extreme obesity	>40	III

Data from National Heart, Lung, and Blood Institute. Clinical guidelines on the identification, evaluation, and treatment of overweight and obesity in adults: the evidence report. Available at: www.nhlbi.nih.gov. Accessed September 17, 2010.

appropriate for an aging population and these changes in height and lean body and fat mass vary not only by age and gender but also by race/ethnic background.[4]

The history of defining sarcopenia has its genesis with Baumgartner and colleagues,[5] who used an approach analogous to the BMI to index relative skeletal muscle mass (SMM). They used appendicular SMM (ASM) from DXA and adjusted for height because of the strong association between height and appendicular lean body mass. The ASM divided by height squared (ASM/m²) formed a relative skeletal muscle index (RSMI). Using principles similar to defining osteoporosis, low RSMI (sarcopenia) was defined as less than 2 SD from the mean of a young reference population.[6] The resulting cut scores to define sarcopenia were less than 7.26 kg/m² for men and less than 5.45 kg/m² for women.[5] Lau and colleagues[7] used the same method and developed cut scores for the Asian population. A few years later, Janssen and colleagues[8] developed the second definition of sarcopenia using bioelectrical impedance (BIA) data from a young reference group in the Third National Health and Nutrition Examination Survey (NHANES III). The BIA data were used to predict total SMM. SMM (kg) was expressed 2 ways to create index SMM: (1) as a percentage of total body weight and (2) divided by height squared, similar to RSMI. A criticism of the first index was that the ratio of whole-body SMM divided by body weight is dependent on body fatness and that the variation in body fat is generally greater than that of SMM.[9] The second method resulted in cut scores that were similar to those derived by RSMI, and an SMM index of 5.76 kg/m² to 6.75 kg/m² was classified as class I sarcopenia and 5.75 kg/m² or less as class II sarcopenia in women. Values for men were 8.51 kg/m² to 10.75 kg/m² for class I and 8.50 kg/m² or less as class II. An important addition was that Janssen and associates calibrated these cut scores against prevalent disability using receiver operating characteristic analysis rather than basing them on a reference population. Concurrently, Newman and colleagues[10] proposed a method that used both body height and total body fat to adjust ASM using regression methods. The lowest 20th percentile of the residuals of regression models of body height and total body fat on ASM produced cut scores that provided similar classification to the RSMI.

The European Working Group on Sarcopenia in Older People (EWGSOP) recently published a practical clinical definition and consensus diagnostic criteria for age-related sarcopenia.[11] It was proposed that for a diagnosis of sarcopenia both low muscle mass and low muscle function (either strength or performance) must be present. EWGSOP argued that defining sarcopenia using only muscle mass was too narrow and likely of limited clinical value. This may be a reasonable argument in that the relationship between muscle mass and function is nonlinear. Furthermore, it was also argued that a new term, dynapenia, was unwarranted because sarcopenia has only recently become a more widely recognized term and changing the terminology could lead to further confusion.[12] The EWGSOP also proposed categories and stages of sarcopenia from presarcopenia to severe sarcopenia. Presarcopenia presents as only low muscle mass, whereas severe sarcopenia involves low muscle mass coupled with low muscular strength and functional performance. In the clinical setting, EWGSOP proposed BIA as a portable and inexpensive alternative to DXA and that muscle strength could be measured by grip strength and physical performance using the Short Physical Performance Battery that includes measures of balance, gait, and muscular strength and endurance.[11]

Sarcopenic obesity, or the combination of low lean body mass and high fat mass, was originally defined using an operational definition of sarcopenia as less than 2 SD below the gender-specific young reference group, with total percentage body fat greater than 27% in men and greater than 38% in women, although other definitions have been proposed.[13] Davison and colleagues[14] defined sarcopenic obese individuals in the upper 2 quintiles of body fat and lower third of muscle mass. Newman and colleagues[10] used ASM relative to height and total fat mass computed from residuals of a linear regression model. Using this strategy, persons with a BMI greater than 30 kg/m² were not classified as sarcopenic using Baumgartner's RSMI, whereas 11.5% of men and 14.4% of obese women were defined as sarcopenic using the residuals method. They concluded that the definition proposed by Baumgartner may underestimate sarcopenia in overweight and obese persons, leading to an overall underestimation of sarcopenic obesity.[10] The prevalence of these body composition phenotypes in the context of these differing views and approaches on classification criteria is discussed later. **Table 2** provides a summary of the differences in body composition components across the 4 body composition phenotypes.

PREVALENCE OF SARCOPENIA, OBESITY, AND SARCOPENIC OBESITY

The errors introduced using BMI to categorize obesity and the lack of consensus on how to define sarcopenia have hampered efforts to accurately determine prevalence of these body composition phenotypes. There is evidence that the prevalence of obesity and sarcopenic obesity is rising and may also vary across different populations.

Sarcopenia Prevalence Data

In a cohort of Hispanic and non-Hispanic white older adults, the prevalence of sarcopenia using DXA increased from 15% in those between 60 and 69 years to 40% in those over 80 regardless of body fatness.[15] These estimates were later recognized as positively biased, possibly due to the use of BIA to predict ASM in some participants. In a large healthy cohort of 1700 community-dwelling older adults using BMI, BIA, and Baumgartner's sarcopenia cut scores, 6.2% of men and 5.9% of women

Table 2
Body composition phenotype characteristics

	Sarcopenic	Obese	Sarcopenic Obese
Weight	Low	High	Normal
Fat Mass	Low/normal	High	High
SMM	Low	Normal/high	Low
BMI (kg/m²)	Low	High	Normal
Waist Circumference	Low/normal	High	Normal/high

Abbreviations: BMI, body mass index; SMM, skeletal muscle mass.

were sarcopenic, increasing with age to 16% of men and 13% of women by age 85.[16] In another large US cohort (Health, Aging, and Body Composition [Health ABC] Study), 2984 participants were assessed by DXA and 2 methods were applied to classify sarcopenia.[10] The methods used were Baumgartner's cut scores, and appendicular lean mass adjusted for height and body fat mass from residuals. Using either method, participants in the lowest 20th percentile were classified as sarcopenic. Conversely, the prevalence of sarcopenia in overweight and obese groups using Baumgartner's cut scores were 8.9% and 0%, respectively. Using residuals, the percentages were 15.4% and 11.5% for men and 21.7% and 21% for women, respectively. The results were similar when using percentage body fat to define overweight. Estrada and colleagues[17] found similar differences when using either the RSMI approach or ASM/body mass in 189 healthy, nonobese, white, postmenopausal women on hormone replacement therapy. Using the RSMI approach, 25.9% were classified as sarcopenic. This method identified sarcopenia in 36.7% of lean women but only 9.2% in overweight women and none in obese women. When they applied the ASM adjusted for body mass rather than height in m^2,[2] 8.5% of lean women were classified as sarcopenic, but 40% of overweight women and 85.7% of obese women were classified as sarcopenic. Iannuzzi-Sucich and colleagues[18] obtained DXA on 337 older women and men and using RSMI, the prevalence of sarcopenia was 22.6% in women and 26.8% in men. Using the NHANES III data set and applying the RSMI calculated from BIA, they found 10% of US women and 7% of men aged older than 60 were severely sarcopenic.[19]

There have been several large European cohort studies investigating the prevalence of sarcopenia. The EPIDOS cohort used RSMI from DXA and reported on 2 studies involving more than 1300 older French community-dwelling women. The prevalence of sarcopenia increased with age from 8.9% at 76 to 80 years to 10.9% at 86 to 95 years.[20,21] Tichet and coworkers[22] derived a muscle mass index (MMI) from BIA in a French population and reported 2.8% of women and 3.6% of men were sarcopenic, but this increased to 23.6% (women) and 12.5% (men) using RSMI. They suggested that MMI and skeletal muscle index (SMI) identified different sarcopenic populations, leaner with MMI and fatter with SMI. In a cohort of more than 1000 community-dwelling older Italians, a CT scan of the calf cross-sectional area was used to assess sarcopenia. It was reported that 20% of men were sarcopenic at 65 years and up to 70% at 85 years, with 5% and 15%, respectively, of women.[23] A smaller study in Germany (n = 110) used body cell mass from BIA and reported that 22% of men and 20% of women were classified as sarcopenic.[24] Using lean body mass from BIA identified only 4% of men and 11% of women as sarcopenic. A study of older Italian women after hip surgery (n = 313)[25] reported 58% were sarcopenic using DXA and ASM/m^2.[25]

In Asia and the Pacific regions, a study of older Taiwanese (n = 302)[26] reported 18.6% of women and 23.6% of men were sarcopenic using BIA and Janssen's cut scores.[26] A larger study in Hong Kong (262 men and 265 women), using DXA and ASM/m^2 cut scores and their own healthy young (20–50 years) reference group, reported 7.6% of women and 12.3% of men were sarcopenic.[7] A sample of 526 Korean adults using DXA and ASM/m^2 reported that 6.3% of men and 4.1% of women were sarcopenic.[27] Using the residuals method in this same sample, 15.4% of men and 22.3% of women were sarcopenic. In a small study of 183 older European New Zealanders, DXA and ASM/m^2 classified 12% of women and 4% of men as sarcopenic.[28]

Obesity Prevalence Data

BMI from either direct measure or self-report is widely used to classify older adults as overweight or obese. As discussed previously, however, loss of height and relative increase in body fat with age make this measure prone to systematic misclassification error. The prevalence of obesity in older adults appears to be increasing in most developed nations of the world. A review by Villareal and colleagues[29] summarized several large population-based cross-sectional studies, primarily in the United States, that showed body weight and BMI gradually increase during adult life, peaking at 50 to 59 years in both men and women and then tending to decrease after age 60. Longitudinal studies indicate, however, only a small decrease in obesity prevalence in older adults over the age 60. In a US survey, the prevalence of obesity was 22.9% in 60 to 69 year olds and 15.5% in those older than 70, representing a 56% and 36% increase, respectively, from 1991 prevalence data.[30,31] Trends may be slightly lower in parts of Europe, where 22% of woman and 12% of men older than 75 are reportedly obese and there seems to be geographic variation, with Central, Eastern, and Southern Europe having higher rates of obesity than in Western and Northern Europe.[32–34] Data from a 1996 to 1997 survey on 13,000 older Canadians reported that 39% and 13% were classified as overweight and obese, respectively, and newer statistics mirror the situation in the United States.[35] Using similar methodology in rural and urban communities in Mexico, 20.9% of the older population were obese and the prevalence decreased with age.[36] Using BMI to measure obesity, 95% of Pacific men and 100% of Pacific women in New Zealand between the ages of 35 and 74 were overweight or obese, and older Pacific adults were 11 times more likely to be obese than their Europeans counterparts.[37] In the smaller study of older European New Zealanders, DXA cut scores of 40% body fat for women and 30% body fat for men classified 46% of women and 47% of men as obese.[28]

Sarcopenic Obesity Prevalence Data

The previous sections discussed the challenges of using BMI, RSMI, and other indices to classify older adults as obese or sarcopenic. An even greater challenge is to identify sarcopenic obese older adults where the combination of low lean body and higher fat mass can result in normal or near normal body weight and BMI. Currently, DXA is considered the gold standard for assessing sarcopenic obesity, but there is a paucity of prevalence data. Using Baumgartner's cut scores in an older New Mexican cohort, the prevalence of sarcopenic obesity was approximately 2% in those 60 to 69 years old increasing to approximately 10% in those 80 and older.[15] Using a definition of the upper 2 quintiles of body fat with the lower 3 quintiles of muscle mass, 3 studies reported the prevalence of sarcopenic obesity as approximately 10% in men and approximately 7% to 12% in women.[14,38,39] Newman and colleagues,[10] applying both residual and RSMI approaches, found that 8.9% of overweight men and 7.1% of overweight women were sarcopenic obese using RSMI, whereas the residuals method classified 15.4% of men and 21.7% of women, respectively as sarcopenic obese. Kim and colleagues[27] applied several approaches—RSMI, lower quintiles of SMI and total body fat, and their new index of SMI plus 2 higher quintiles of percentage total body fat—to determine the prevalence of sarcopenic obesity in older Korean adults.[27] They reported that 1.3% of men and 0.8% of women were sarcopenic obese using RSMI, whereas using their own index 5.1% of men and 12.5% of women were sarcopenic obese. Thus, as for sarcopenia and obesity, the reported prevalence of sarcopenic obesity varies considerably across study populations even when similar methods are applied. Several concerns should be noted. There are few, if any, systematic evaluations of the relative sensitivity and specificity of these various methods. More large-scale investigations applying these different approaches to the same study sample are needed to address this question. The relative precision and validity of the various measurement methods warrants careful consideration, particularly for sarcopenia. BIA is considerably less precise than DXA or imaging methods, and measures of muscle strength and physical performance in elders can be confounded by morbidity (eg, arthritis and neuromuscular disease) and volition. The use of 2 or more methods can lead to compounding measurement errors and an increased likelihood of misclassification. It has been debated whether the definition put forth by Baumgartner underestimates sarcopenia in overweight and obese persons.[40] If body fatness influences the identification of sarcopenia from certain methods, then prevalence estimates will vary across population samples depending on the average of level of obesity.

ETIOLOGY OF BODY COMPOSITION CHANGES WITH AGING

There is a growing body of evidence that the loss of muscle mass and strength (sarcopenia) during aging is a complex interplay of factors, including physical activity, neuromuscular changes, hormones (insulin, testosterone/estrogen, growth hormone [GH]/insulinlike growth factor 1 [IGF-1], vitamin D, and parathyroid hormone), proinflammatory cytokines, oxidative stress, mitochondrial dysfunction, apoptosis pathways, genetics, dietary energy and protein intake, and other factors yet to be identified. It is beyond the scope of this review to discuss in detail each of the factors and their individual roles in the development and progression of sarcopenia. This topic has been the focus of many reviews: several published between 2000 and 2010 are listed in **Table 3** and in the reference list.[32,34,41–75]

There are few published investigations on the etiology of sarcopenic obesity. The development of obesity, however, may play a role in sarcopenic obesity, as discussed later. The previous section documented evidence that in developed and some rapidly developing countries obesity prevalence is increasing even into old age.[29,76] Obesity is largely the result of an imbalance between energy intake and expenditure, which may worsen with age.[29] A recent review[77] concluded that during aging reductions in the mass of individual organs and tissues contribute to a reduction in resting metabolic rate.[78] Resting metabolic rate makes up approximately 70% of total energy expenditure, with physical activity contributing approximately 20% and thermic effect of foods approximately 10% to total energy expenditure.[22,29] A decreasing resting metabolic rate could lead to changes in body composition that favor increasing fat mass.

In concert with these changes, there is growing evidence that adipose tissue not only is a storage depot for excess energy but also acts as an endocrine organ secreting a variety of adipokines, some of which have proinflammatory actions that have an impact on various metabolic functions.[78] As obesity develops, the adipocytes enlarge and undergo molecular and cellular changes, resulting in increased fasting circulating levels of whole-body free fatty acids and glycerol that are believed to promote insulin resistance.[79] The second effect is the production of inflammatory cytokines, such as interleukin (IL)-1, IL-6, and tumor necrosis factor α (TNF-α).[80–82] Macrophage numbers in adipose tissue increase with obesity and are responsible for the secretion of some of these proinflammatory cytokines, in particular IL-6 and TNF-α, but other molecules, such as leptin (proinflammatory) and adiponectin (anti-inflammatory), are produced directly by adipocytes. Taken together these adipocytokines are also associated with the development of insulin resistance.[80,83] It has been proposed that the chronic inflammatory state induced by obesity drives the progressive loss of muscle mass[38,40] that ultimately leads to sarcopenic obesity by upregulation of protein degradation via the ubiquitin-proteasome pathway. There are also changes in fat distribution with increases in waist circumference and visceral fat with decreases in subcutaneous fat.[38] Roubenoff[84] proposed that the production of TNF-α and leptin influences not only insulin resistance but also energy metabolism and GH secretion, which could additionally drive the loss of muscle and increased fat deposition. It has also been postulated that the fatty infiltration of muscle that occurs in obesity may drive the inflammatory environment in muscle, more so than muscle that does not have fatty infiltration.[40] In a highly inflammatory state, obese people prefentially mobilize muscle, not fat,[61] and this represents a major contributor to fat gain, which in turn reinforces muscle loss.[63] This creates a vicious cycle of fat gain and muscle loss, which could lead to greater loss of muscle and function (as shown in **Fig. 1**). If future investigations consistently confirm this finding, it may be a biologically plausible mechanism. It also raises the question of what the true prevalence of sarcopenic obesity will be in the future if longevity continues to increase.

FUNCTIONAL AND METABOLIC CONSEQUENCES OF SARCOPENIA, OBESITY, AND SARCOPENIC OBESITY

Investigations into the consequences and correlates of sarcopenia have largely focused on changes in the neuromuscular system and the subsequent loss of function. Basal metabolic rate, immune function, regulation of body temperature and blood glucose, and the preservation of internal organs, nerves, and blood vessels all depend, however, on the maintenance of skeletal muscle.[85] It was previously thought that the sarcopenic process was the same regardless of whether this was pure sarcopenia or sarcopenic obesity, but, as discussed previously, the growing understanding of the intimate communication between adipose and muscle tissues may challenge this earlier thinking. This section begins with a discussion of sarcopenia, then discusses obesity, and finally addresses sarcopenic obesity.

The primary functional consequence of sarcopenia is the loss of muscle strength and power, which may eventually lead to mobility dysfunction and increased risk for falls. The recommended definition of sarcopenia as the presence of both the loss of muscle mass and function recognizes this relationship. Cross-sectional and longitudinal studies, however, have produced conflicting results. Rolland[20] obtained DXA and grip strength from a large cross-section of women over 70 years old in the EPIDOS trial (n = 1458). When sarcopenia was defined using SMM, they found no association between sarcopenia and falls or functional deficits. When sarcopenia was defined using ASM/m^2, however, there was an association with more difficulties of instrumental activities of daily living (IADLs). Data from the Health ABC Study cohort (n = 2631, age 70–79)[86] reported that those with the lowest muscle mass were more likely to develop mobility limitations but that low muscle strength showed a stronger relationship. A later study from this cohort (n = 3075) reported that body fat and leg strength, rather than muscle mass, were independent determinants of lower-extremity performance.[87] Similarly, Goodpaster and colleagues,[88] reporting on data from this same cohort (n = 1880), described that the loss of muscle mass was associated with a decrease in strength but that the loss of strength was more rapid than that of muscle mass. They suggested that muscle quality was playing a larger role in associations with muscle function. The a clinico-epidemiologic study in the Chianti area (Tuscany, Italy) cohort (n = 1030) used anthropometric measures and reported that age-related mobility declines were related to the loss of strength and power in the lower body.[23] Data from the Cardiovascular Health Study (n = 5036)[89] used BIA measures and reported that the likelihood of disability was greatest in only those with severe sarcopenia and not milder forms. A longitudinal study in Sweden (NORA)[90] in a smaller cohort (n = 323) that also used BIA measures reported that maintaining fat-free mass was important for maintaining functional abilities during aging.[90] A large study (n = 4000) of community-dwelling Chinese older adults reported

Table 3
Review publications on the etiology of sarcopenia listed chronologically 2000–2010

Author(s), Reference Number (Year)	Publication Type	Primary Mechanisms Discussed
Roubenoff and Hughes,[41] 2000	Review	Inflammatory cytokines, physical activity, central nervous system, sex hormones, GH, insulin action, protein intake, anabolic stimuli
Roubenoff,[42] 2000	Review	Central nervous system, muscle contractility, GH, inflammatory cytokines, physical activity
Morley et al,[43] 2001	Review	Muscle fibers, protein synthesis, inflammatory cytokines, anorexia, physical activity, motor units
Roubenoff,[44] 2001	Review	Central nervous system, muscle contractility, humoral factors (GH, sex hormones, and inflammatory cytokines), physical activity
Bales and Ritchie,[45] 2002	Review	Appetite, nutritional deficiency, weight loss, inflammatory cytokines
Leeuwenburgh,[46] 2003	Brief review	Apoptotic cell death. Calcium and hydrogen peroxide as key signals
Doherty,[32] 2003	Review	Decreasing motor units, muscle fibers type, anorexia, protein intake, GH, testosterone, HRT, inflammatory cytokines physical activity
Marcell,[47] 2003	Review	Physical activity, protein metabolism, hormonal, inflammatory cytokines, gene expression, denervation, apoptosis
Greenlund and Nair,[48] 2003	Discussion article	Protein synthesis, mitochondrial dysfunction, anabolic hormones (GH, IGF-1, testosterone, and DHEA), muscle perfusion, neuromuscular changes
Roubenoff,[34] 2003	Review	Muscle quality, α motor units, GH, testosterone/estrogen, inflammatory cytokines, protein intake, proteasome activity, physical activity
Evans,[49] 2004	Review	Dietary protein, physical activity
Fulle et al,[50] 2004	Hypothesis article	ROS sarcoplasmic reticulum
Borst,[51] 2004	Review	Testosterone, HRT, GH therapy, high-intensity resistance training
Dupont-Versteegden,[52] 2005	Discussion article	Apoptosis pathways
Dirks and Leeuwenburgh,[53] 2005	Review	Mitochondrial dysfunction, oxidative stress, apoptosis
Kamen,[54] 2005	Review	Neural factors—motor recruitment, rate coding, motor unit synchronization, neuromuscular adaptations to resistance training
Solomon and Bouloux,[55] 2006	Review	Calcium, vitamin D, glucocorticoids, GH, IGFs and isoforms, androgens, myostatin
Faulkner et al,[56] 2007	Review	Motor units, muscle atrophy, frailty, master athlete records
Sayers,[57] 2007	Review	Life course model, developmental plasticity, birth weight and grip strength, environmental influences

Study	Type	Topics
Semba et al,[58] 2007	Minireview	Carotenoids protective against oxidative stress
Roubenoff,[59] 2007	Review	Inflammatory cytokines, regular physical activity
Chahal and Drake,[60] 2007	Review	Estrogen and testosterone, serum concentrations of GH, IGF-1, and dehydroepiandrosterone and its sulfate-bound form
Jensen,[61] 2008	Workshop notes	Inflammatory cytokines, apoptosis ROS mtDNA deletions
Paddon-Jones et al,[62] 2008	Discussion article	Dietary protein, protein quality, renal function
Cesari and Pahor,[63] 2008	Review	Demographic factors, race/ethnicity, physical activity, nutrition, smoking, inflammatory cytokines, testosterone, GH
Johnston et al,[64] 2008	Symposium	Mitochondrial DNA deletions, electron transport chain, ROS, resistance training
Hiona and Leeuwenburgh,[65] 2008	Minireview	Mitochondrial DNA mutations, ROS, electron transport system
Rolland et al,[67] 2008	Review	Physical activity, neuromuscular, endocrine (insulin, testosterone/estrogen, GH/IGF-1, vitamin D, parathyroid hormone, proinflammatory cytokines, mitochondrial dysfunction, apoptosis, genetics, diet/protein intake
Boirie,[66] 2009	Discussion article	GH/IGF-1 testosterone, insulin resistance. Inflammatory cytokines, protein intake/impaired protein metabolism, exercise
Huang and Hood,[68] 2009	Critical review	Mitochondria
Snijders et al,[69] 2009	Review	Skeletal muscle satellite cells, myonuclei, structural changes in myofibers
Paddon-Jones and Rasmussen,[70] 2009	Review	Dietary protein, leucine supplementation, physical activity
Lang et al,[71] 2010	Review	Muscle fiber structure, neuromuscular function, contractile proteins, neurodegeneration, protein balance, IGF-1, inflammatory cytokines, oxidative damage, muscle-tendon system
Meng and Yu,[72] 2010	Review	Oxidative stress, ROS, modulation of transcription factors, proinflammatory cytokines, mtDNA damage, proapoptosis factors, apoptosis
Marzetti et al,[73] 2010	Review	Mitochondrial dysfunction, iron accumulation, mitochondrial-mediated apoptosis
Aagaard et al,[74] 2010	Review	Loss of spinal motor neurons secondary to apoptosis, reduced IGF-1, proinflamatory cytokines, oxidative stress
Kim et al,[75] 2010	Review	Dietary protein, amino acids, protein quality, leucine metabolism, oxidative stress, antioxidant supplementation

Abbreviations: DHEA, dehydroepiandrosterone; GH, growth hormone; HRT, hormone replacement therapy; IFG-1, insulin-like growth factor; mtDNA, mitochondrial DNA; ROS, reactive oxygen species.

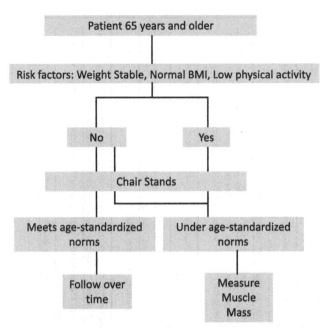

Fig. 1. Algorithm to clinically assess sarcopenic-obesity.

that sarcopenia was associated with physical inactivity[91] and a smaller study (n = 275) reported that the association between sarcopenia and physical disability was largely mediated by cardiopulmonary fitness, which was related to physical activity. Sarcopenia has been reported in physically trained older persons, however, and even elite athletes lose muscle mass and function over time despite continued training.[92] In a small sub study of the New Mexico Aging Process Study, highly active older sarcopenic adults were age and sex matched to equally active adults with normal lean body and fat mass. Muscle energetics during exercise was measured using ^{31}P magnetic resonance spectroscopy and mildly impaired muscle energetics was detected in the sarcopenic group.[93] Finally, there may be a gender interaction in the association between muscle mass and function. Although men have greater SMM and limb power than women, the percentage of age-related functional losses are similar between the genders over a life-time, whereas absolute losses are greater in men.[71]

Sarcopenia has been reported as predictive of hospital-acquired infections in frail older patients, which could have implications for mortality.[94] Data from the Health ABC Study[95] reported, however, that although lower muscle strength was linked to mortality, this could not be attributed to sarcopenia per se because controlling for muscle size measured by DXA did not attenuate the associations.[95] The development of sarcopenia is driven by multiple factors, as highlighted in **Table 3**, and it is associated with the loss of muscle power and function.

In addition to functional disability, other well-known health sequelae, such as cardiovascular disease, metabolic syndrome (combination of higher insulin/blood glucose, hypertension, and dislipidemia), osteoarthritis, pulmonary abnormalities, some forms of cancer, and increased risk of chronic inflammation, are associated with obesity. Each of these have been discussed in comprehensive reviews and even accounting for these factors, the relationship between obesity and functional disability remains intact.[29,38,76,96]

Alley and Chang,[97] using data from the NHANES III and NHANES IV, reported that rates of cardiovascular disease have improved in obese elders, most likely due to improvements in medical care. Despite these improvements, there has been no similar reduction in functional disability. To the contrary, the group surveyed in NHANES IV (1999–2004) was more likely to report functional impairments than those in the NHANES III. Moreover, reductions in IADL impairment in nonobese older individuals were not reported by those who were obese. It was suggested that developing obesity at a younger age could lead to an increased burden of disability in older obese populations, in those who survive into old age. This was confirmed in the Established Populations for Epidemiologic Studies of the Elderly, which reported overweight and obese older adults are living longer but spending more years of their life with some disability than leaner counterparts.[98] It has also been suggested that studies investigating obesity and disability need to consider the role of weight history and periods of weight gain and duration of obesity to more accurately assess this relationship.[99] **Table 4** summarizes some larger cohort and cross-sectional studies since 2000 that have specifically investigated obesity and disability.[14,86,87,97,100–107]

Identifying consequences associated with sarcopenic obesity poses many challenges because a consensus regarding the development and identification of this body composition phenotype has not been established. Given that BMI and weight cannot detect a sarcopenic-obese phenotype, it is likely that its effect on mortality and morbidity is underestimated.[38] Baumgartner[13] first described the consequences of sarcopenic obesity in an older New Mexican population, which demonstrated lower grip strength and greater functional impairment in the sarcopenic obese compared with both obese and sarcopenic participants. Longitudinal data from the New Mexico Aging Process Study reported that the sarcopenic obese were 2.5 times more likely to report IADL disability over a 5-year follow up, regardless of comorbidity.[108] The prevalence of metabolic syndrome was greatest in the nonsarcopenic obese, followed by sarcopenic obese, and lowest in the sarcopenic. This data agrees with Aubertin-Leheudre and colleagues,[109,110] who reported that obese women had significantly more fat-free mass, abdominal fat mass, and visceral fat mass and a worse lipid profile than sarcopenic obese postmenopausal women, although this cohort was younger than the New Mexico cohort. As part of the Korean Longitudinal Study on Health and Aging, the relationship between sarcopenic obesity and metabolic syndrome was investigated.[75] The prevalence of sarcopenic obesity was low, particularly in women when classified using ASM/m^2 (16.7% of men and 5.7% of women); however, when adjusting ASM for weight, the prevalence rose to 35.1% and 48.1% in men and women, respectively. Using the homeostasis model assessment of insulin resistance, participants with sarcopenic obesity were 8 times as likely to develop metabolic syndrome compared with the obese or sarcopenic groups. This question also was examined in the Cardiovascular Health Study using data at baseline and at 8-year follow up.[111] Participants were classified as sarcopenic obese based on waist circumference and either muscle mass (by BIA) or muscle strength. When using muscle mass and waist circumference, cardiovascular disease risk was not significantly elevated. When using muscle strength and waist circumference, risk was increased 23%. They concluded that muscle strength might be more important than muscle mass for cardiovascular disease protection during aging.

As discussed previously, proinflammatory cytokines are believed involved in the development and progression of sarcopenic obesity and may be associated with muscle dysfunction. Furthermore, Alzheimer disease, atherosclerosis, diabetes, and even cancer have inflammatory components, and if the vicious cycle exists in sarcopenic obesity as it does in obesity, these diseases may also develop in sarcopenic

Table 4
Obesity and disability investigations listed chronologically 2000–2010

Author(s), Reference Number (Year)	Study Design (Sample Size)	Gender(s) and Age	Body Composition, Method, and Outcome Measures	Main Findings
Visser et al,[86] 2005	Cohort, Health ABC (n = 2579)	M & W 70–79 years	DXA, chair stand, leg strength	Higher body fat was associated with poor lower-extremity performance. Body fat and leg strength were independent determinates of lower-extremity performance.
Friedmann et al,[99] 2001	Cross-sectional (n = 7120)	M & W 65–98 years	BMI, self-report function	Women had higher rates of functional limitations within all BMI groups than men. BMI at which risk increases is lower for women than for men.
Davison et al,[14] 2002	Cross-sectional (n = 2917)	M & W 70 years and older	Skinfold and BIA estimated body fat and muscle mass, mobility-related functional limitations	High-percentage body fat and high BMI were associated with greater functional limitations in women. Relationship was not clear in men.
Sternfeld et al,[101] 2002	Cross-section of cohort (n = 1655)	M&W 55 years and older	BIA, self-report physical function, walking speed, grip strength	Fat mass has negative impact on physical performance, whereas the impact of lean mass was not as significant in absolute terms but was important relative to body fat.
Jensen and Friedmann,[118] 2002	Cohort, Geisinger Health Plan (n = 2634)	M & W 65 years and older	BMI, self-report ADL, IADL	Obesity was a risk factor for functional decline in older persons, in particular women. Ten-pound weight loss and 20-pound weight gain were risk factors for functional decline.
Newman et al,[102] 2003	Cohort, Health ABC Study (n = 2623)	M & W 70–79 years	DXA, upper and lower strength, muscle quality, self-report physical activity	Lower muscle quality in obese may mediate association between body fat and lower physical function.
Villareal et al,[103] 2004	Matched cross-sectional (n = 157)	M & W 65 years and older	DXA, physical performance test, exercise stress test, lower-extremity strength, gait speed, static and dynamic balance	Physical frailty was associated with low fat-free mass, poor muscle quality, and lower quality of life.

Study	Study design (n)	Population	Measures	Findings
Rolland et al,[104] 2004	Cross-sectional (n = 1454)	Women older than 70 years	DXA, grip strength, and leg strength	Muscle strength adjusted for muscle mass was not associated with obesity. In active women, low limb strength increased with increasing BMI.
Zoico et al,[39] 2004	Cross-sectional (n = 167)	Women 67–78 years 20–50 years (reference group)	BMI, DXA, self-report ADL, leg strength	High body fat and BMI were associated with functional limitations. Only SMI predicted functional impairment and disability. Isometric leg strength was lower in sarcopenia and sarcopenic obesity.
Visser et al,[86] 2005	Cohort, Health ABC (n = 3075)	M & W 70–79 years	DXA chair stand, leg strength	Higher body fat was associated with poorer performance (stronger association in women than in men). Body fat and leg muscle strength (not mass) were independent determinants of lower-extremity performance in both genders.
Alley and Chang,[97] 2007	Cross-sectional NHANES III and IV (n = 10,708)	M & W 60 years and older	BMI, self-report ability/disability	Obese participants in more recent data collection were more likely to report reductions in ADL.
Stenholm et al,[105] 2009	Cohort, InCHIANTI (n = 930)	M & W 65 years and older	BMI, self-report function, walking speed, leg strength	Older obese adults with low muscle strength have higher risk for decline of walking speed, and for the development of new disability.
Rolland et al,[106] 2009	Cross-sectional from cohort study EPIDOS (n = 1308)	Women 75 years and older	DXA, self-report physical function	Obesity was associated with difficulty with physical function with or without sarcopenia. Sarcopenia was only associated with physical function difficulty in the presence of obesity.
Bouchard et al,[107] 2009	Cohort (NuAge) (n = 894)	M & W 65 year and older	DXA, BMI, timed up and go, chair stand, walking speed, one leg stand, global physical capacity score	Obesity seemed to contribute more to lower physical capacity than sarcopenia.

Abbreviations: ADL, activities of daily living; M & W, men and women.

obese individuals, bearing in mind that disease progression is likely dependent on individual genetic backgrounds.[112,113]

There are few studies that have directly measured physical function in older adults with sarcopenic obesity. Baumgartner and colleagues[13,108] were among the first to report that sarcopenic obesity predicted IADL disability as well as gait and balance disorders. Objectively measured function and body composition in a small New Zealand study also reported functional deficits in people with sarcopenic obesity.[93] Zoico and colleagues[39] could only find a trend toward an increased risk in functional impairment in sarcopenic-obese women. Conversely, a Canadian study did not find lower physical capacity in sarcopenic-obese men and women, whereas data from the Health ABC Study cohort[102] reported that both high body fat and low body fat have adverse effects on both muscle strength and muscle quality.[102,107] Two cross-sectional studies also did not find an association between sarcopenic obesity and physical function.[14,39] Differences in the measurement and definitions of sarcopenic obesity may partially explain these conflicting results, and a definition that considers both obesity and muscle weakness has been proposed.[105] Two recent studies directly measured the biomechanics and gait characteristics of obese and sarcopenic-obese postmenopausal women.[114,115] Increased plantar pressure was found in both obese women and sarcopenic obese women and higher loading in the stance phase in sarcopenic-obese women compared with women with normal body composition. The temporal characteristics of foot rollover during walking were also altered in the sarcopenic-obese women. These findings could have implications for gait and balance deficits or discomfort while walking.

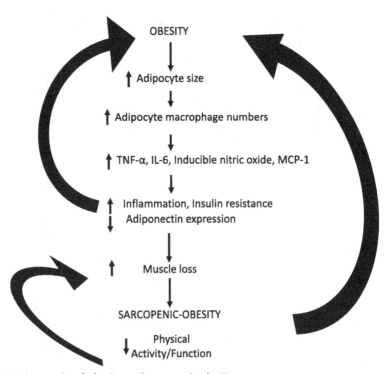

Fig. 2. Vicious cycle of obesity and sarcopenic-obesity.

Larger, longitudinal studies and standardized definitions of obesity and sarcopenia are needed to resolve these conflicting results. With a few exceptions, the majority of studies have been cross-sectional and cannot define the causal direction of observed associations between these body composition phenotypes and correlates, such as disability and morbidity. Reliance on DXA-measured body composition to identify sarcopenic obesity may present a challenge in some clinical settings. The authors proposed an algorithm similar to that published by Cruz-Jentoft and colleageus[11] and one currently being developed by Manini and Clark for dynapenia.[116] The algorithm in **Fig. 2** assumes support for the evidence that physical function is compromised in the sarcopenic obese phenotype, while acknowledging the literature is conflicting.

SUMMARY

There is compelling evidence that aging populations are living longer but with greater disability, and as a result the prevalence of sarcopenia, obesity, and sarcopenic obesity will increase. There are no published studies to date that have investigated if long-standing obesity eventually leads to sarcopenic obesity in the longest-lived adults, and what implications there may be for physical function and other health outcomes. If obese people with weak lower-extremity muscles are the most functionally impaired, it can only be surmised that function worsens as the loss of lean mass accelerates in older age. A recent systematic review by Moreland and colleagues[117] reported that older adults with lower-body weakness were up to 2.5 more likely to fall (odds ratio 1.2–2.5), and the risk increased to up to 9 times (odds ratio 2.2–9.9) for recurrent falls, a grim statistic given the high rate of hip fractures and poor health outcomes after a fall. The data cited in this review also point to the need for investigations into the joint relationships of obesity, muscle mass, and composition with muscle function and the need to pursue simple and cost-effective clinical assessments to identify these body composition phenotypes. Until a greater understanding of these complex relationships is reached, individual-level preventive measures to slow functional decline regardless of body composition phenotype seem warranted, although ideally primary or secondary prevention of undesirable body composition phenotypes and loss of function is more desirable.

ACKNOWLEDGMENTS

A special thank you to Aimee Ward, MPH, for her significant contribution in the preparation of this manuscript.

REFERENCES

1. Villareal DT, Shah K. Obesity in older adults—a growing problem. In: Bales CW, Ritchie CS, editors. Nutrition and health: handbook of clinical nutrition and aging. 2nd edition. New York: Humana Press; 2009. p. 263–77.
2. Ritz P. Obesity in the elderly: should we be using new diagnostic criteria? J Nutr Health Aging 2009;13(3):168–9.
3. Abellan Van Kan G. Epidemiology and consequences of sarcopenia. J Nutr Health Aging 2009;13(8):708–12.
4. Han SS, Kim KW, Kim KI, et al. Lean mass index: a better predictor of mortality than body mass index in elderly Asians. J Am Geriatr Soc 2010;58(2):312–7.
5. Baumgartner RN, Koehler KM, Gallagher D, et al. Epidemiology of sarcopenia among the elderly in New Mexico. Am J Epidemiol 1998;147(8):755–63.

6. Mott JW, Wang JC, Thornton DB, et al. Relationship between body fat and age in 4 ethnic groups. Am J Clin Nutr 1999;69:1007–13.

7. Lau EM, Lynn HS, Woo JW, et al. Prevalence of and risk factors for sarcopenia in elderly Chinese men and women. J Gerontol B Psychol Sci Soc Sci 2005;60(2): 213–6.

8. Janssen I, Heymsfield SB, Ross R. Low relative skeletal muscle mass (sarcopenia) in older persons is associated with functional impairment and physical disability. J Am Geriatr Soc 2002;50(5):889–96.

9. Visser M. Towards a definition of sarcopenia—results from epidemiologic studies. J Nutr Health Aging 2009;13(8):713–6.

10. Newman AB, Kupelian V, Visser M, et al. Sarcopenia: alternative definitions and associations with lower extremity function. J Am Geriatr Soc 2003;51(11):1602–9.

11. Cruz-Jentoft AJ, Baeyens JP, Bauer JM, et al. Sarcopenia: European consensus on definition and diagnosis: report of the European Working Group on Sarcopenia in Older People. Age Ageing 2010;39(4):412–23.

12. Clark BC, Manini TM. Sarcopenia =/= dynapenia. J Gerontol A Biol Sci Med Sci 2008;63(8):829–34.

13. Baumgartner RN. Body composition in healthy aging. In Vivo Body Composition Studies. Ann N Y Acad Sci 2000;904:437–48.

14. Davison KK, Ford ES, Cogswell ME, et al. Percentage of body fat and body mass index are associated with mobility limitations in people aged 70 and older from NHANES III. J Am Geriatr Soc 2002;50(11):1802–9.

15. Baumgartner RN. Body composition in healthy aging. Ann N Y Acad Sci 2006; 904(1):437–48.

16. Castillo EM, Goodman-Gruen D, Kritz-Silverstein D, et al. Sarcopenia in elderly men and women - The Rancho Bernardo Study. Am J Prev Med 2003;25(3):226–31.

17. Estrada M, Kleppinger A, Judge JO, et al. Functional impact of relative versus absolute sarcopenia in healthy older women. J Am Geriatr Soc 2007;55(11): 1712–9.

18. Iannuzzi-Sucich M, Prestwood KM, Kenny AM. Prevalence of sarcopenia and predictors of skeletal muscle mass in healthy, older men and women. J Gerontol A Biol Sci Med Sci 2002;57(12):M772–7.

19. Janssen I, Baumgartner RN, Ross R, et al. Skeletal muscle cutpoints associated with elevated physical disability risk in older men and women. Am J Epidemiol 2004;159(4):413–21.

20. Rolland Y. Sarcopenia, calf circumference, and physical function of elderly women: a cross-sectional study. J Am Geriatr Soc 2003;51(8):1120–4.

21. Gillette-Guyonnet S, Nourhashemi F, Andrieu S, et al. Body composition in French women 75+ years of age: the EPIDOS study. Mech Ageing Dev 2003; 124(3):311–6.

22. Tichet J, Vol S, Goxe D, et al. Prevalence of sarcopenia in the French senior population. J Nutr Health Aging 2008;12(3):202–6.

23. Lauretani F, Russo CR, Bandinelli S, et al. Age-associated changes in skeletal muscles and their effect on mobility: an operational diagnosis of sarcopenia. J Appl Physiol 2003;95(5):1851–60.

24. Hedayati KK, Dittmar M. Prevalence of sarcopenia among older community-dwelling people with normal health and nutritional state. Ecol Food Nutr 2010; 49(2):110–28.

25. Di Monaco M, Vallero F, Di Monaco R, et al. Prevalence of sarcopenia and its association with osteoporosis in 313 older women following a hip fracture. Arch Gerontol Geriatr 2011;52(1):71–4.

26. Chien MY, Huang TY, Wu YT. Prevalence of sarcopenia estimated using a bioelectrical impedance analysis prediction equation in community-dwelling elderly people in Taiwan. J Am Geriatr Soc 2008;56(9):1710–5.
27. Kim TN, Yang SJ, Yoo HJ, et al. Prevalence of sarcopenia and sarcopenic obesity in Korean adults: the Korean sarcopenic obesity study. Int J Obes (Lond) 2009;33(8):885–92.
28. Waters DL, Hale L, Grant AM, et al. Osteoporosis and gait and balance disturbances in older sarcopenic obese New Zealanders. Osteoporos Int 2010;21(2): 351–7.
29. Villareal DT, Apovian CM, Kushner RF, et al. Obesity in older adults: technical review and position statement of the American Society for Nutrition and NAASO, The Obesity Society. Obes Res 2005;13(11):1849–63.
30. Flegal KM, Carroll MD, Ogden CL, et al. Prevalence and trends in obesity among US adults, 1999–2000. JAMA 2002;288(14):1723–7.
31. Arterburn DE, Crane PK, Sullivan SD. The coming epidemic of obesity in elderly Americans. J Am Geriatr Soc 2004;52(11):1907–12.
32. Doherty TJ. Aging and sarcopenia. J Appl Physiol 2003;95(4):1717–27.
33. Berghofer A, Pischon T, Reinhold T, et al. Obesity prevalence from a European perspective: a systematic review. BMC Public Health 2008;8:200.
34. Roubenoff R. Sarcopenia: effects on body composition and function. J Gerontol B Psychol Sci Soc Sci 2003;58(11):1012–7.
35. Kaplan MS, Huguet N, Newsom JT, et al. Prevalence and correlates of overweight and obesity among older adults: findings from the Canadian National Population Health Survey. J Gerontol A Biol Sci Med Sci 2003;58(11):1018–30.
36. Ruiz-Arregui L, Castillo-Martinez L, Orea-Tejeda A, et al. Prevalence of self-reported overweight-obesity and its association with socioeconomic and health factors among older Mexican adults. Salud Publica Mex 2007;49(Suppl 4): S482–7.
37. Sundborn G, Metcalf PA, Gentles D, et al. Overweight and obesity prevalence among adult Pacific peoples and Europeans in the Diabetes Heart and Health Study (DHAHS) 2002–2003, Auckland New Zealand. N Z Med J 2010; 123(1311):30–42.
38. Zamboni M, Mazzali G, Zoico E, et al. Health consequences of obesity in the elderly: a review of four unresolved questions. Int J Obes (Lond) 2005;29(9): 1011–29.
39. Zoico E, Di Francesco V, Guralnik JM, et al. Physical disability and muscular strength in relation to obesity and different body composition indexes in a sample of healthy elderly women. Int J Obes Relat Metab Disord 2004; 28(2):234–41.
40. Zamboni M, Mazzali G, Fantin F, et al. Sarcopenic obesity: a new category of obesity in the elderly. Nutr Metab Cardiovasc Dis 2008;18(5):388–95.
41. Roubenoff R, Hughes VA. Sarcopenia: current concepts. J Gerontol A Biol Sci Med Sci 2000;55(12):M716–24.
42. Roubenoff R. Sarcopenia and its implications for the elderly. Eur J Clin Nutr 2000;54:S40–7.
43. Morley JE, Baumgartner RN, Roubenoff R, et al. Sarcopenia. J Lab Clin Med 2001;137(4):231–43.
44. Roubenoff R. Origins and clinical relevance of sarcopenia. Can J Appl Physiol-Revue Canadienne De Physiologie Appliquee 2001;26(1):78–89.
45. Bales CW, Ritchie CS. Sarcopenia, weight loss, and nutritional frailty in the elderly. Annu Rev Nutr 2002;22:309–23.

46. Leeuwenburgh C. Role of apoptosis in sarcopenia. J Gerontol B Psychol Sci Soc Sci 2003;58(11):999–1001.
47. Marcell TJ. Sarcopenia: causes, consequences, and preventions. J Gerontol B Psychol Sci Soc Sci 2003;58(10):911–6.
48. Greenlund LJ, Nair KS. Sarcopenia-consequences, mechanisms, and potential therapies. Mech Ageing Dev 2003;124(3):287–99.
49. Evans WJ. Protein nutrition, exercise and aging. J Am Coll Nutr 2004;23(Suppl 6): 601S–9S.
50. Fulle S, Protasi F, Di Tano G, et al. The contribution of reactive oxygen species to sarcopenia and muscle ageing. Exp Gerontol 2004;39(1):17–24.
51. Borst SE. Interventions for sarcopenia and muscle weakness in older people. Age Ageing 2004;33(6):548–55.
52. Dupont-Versteegden EE. Apoptosis in muscle atrophy: relevance to sarcopenia. Exp Gerontol 2005;40(6):473–81.
53. Dirks AJ, Leeuwenburgh C. The role of apoptosis in age-related skeletal muscle atrophy. Sports Med 2005;35(6):473–83.
54. Kamen G. Aging, resistance training, and motor unit discharge behavior. Can J Appl Physiol-Revue Canadienne De Physiologie Appliquee 2005;30(3):341–51.
55. Solomon AM, Bouloux PM. Modifying muscle mass—the endocrine perspective. J Endocrinol 2006;191(2):349–60.
56. Faulkner JA, Larkin LM, Claflin DR, et al. Age-related changes in the structure and function of skeletal muscles. Clin Exp Pharmacol Physiol 2007;34(11):1091–6.
57. Sayers SP. High-speed power training: a novel approach to resistance training in older men and women. A brief review and pilot study. J Strength Cond Res 2007;21(2):518–26.
58. Semba RD, Lauretani F, Ferrucci L. Carotenoids as protection against sarcopenia in older adults. Arch Biochem Biophys 2007;458(2):141–5.
59. Roubenoff R. Physical activity, inflammation, and muscle loss. Nutr Rev 2007; 65(12 Pt 2):S208–12.
60. Chahal HS, Drake WM. The endocrine system and ageing. J Pathol 2007;211(2): 173–80.
61. Jensen GL. Inflammation: roles in aging and sarcopenia. J Parenter Enteral Nutr 2008;32(6):656–9.
62. Paddon-Jones D, Short KR, Campbell WW, et al. Role of dietary protein in the sarcopenia of aging. Am J Clin Nutr 2008;87(5):1562s–6s.
63. Cesari M, Pahor M. Target population for clinical trials on sarcopenia. J Nutr Health Aging 2008;12(7):470–8.
64. Johnston AP, De Lisio M, Parise G. Resistance training, sarcopenia, and the mitochondrial theory of aging. Appl Physiol Nutr Metab-Physiologie Appliquee Nutrition Et Metabolisme 2008;33(1):191–9.
65. Hiona A, Leeuwenburgh C. The role of mitochondrial DNA mutations in aging and sarcopenia: implications for the mitochondrial vicious cycle theory of aging. Exp Gerontol 2008;43(1):24–33.
66. Boirie Y. Physiopathological mechanism of sarcopenia. J Nutr Health Aging 2009;13(8):717–23.
67. Rolland Y, Czerwinski S, van Kan GA, et al. Sarcopenia: its assessment, etiology, pathogenesis, consequences and future perspectives. J Nutr Health Aging 2008;12(7):433–50.
68. Huang JH, Hood DA. Age-associated mitochondrial dysfunction in skeletal muscle: contributing factors and suggestions for long-term interventions. IUBMB Life 2009;61(3):201–14.

69. Snijders T, Verdijk LB, van Loon LJ. The impact of sarcopenia and exercise training on skeletal muscle satellite cells. Ageing Res Rev 2009;8(4):328–38.
70. Paddon-Jones D, Rasmussen BB. Dietary protein recommendations and the prevention of sarcopenia. Curr Opin Clin Nutr Metab Care 2009;12(1):86–90.
71. Lang T, Streeper T, Cawthon P, et al. Sarcopenia: etiology, clinical consequences, intervention, and assessment. Osteoporos Int 2010;21(4):543–59.
72. Meng SJ, Yu LJ. Oxidative stress, molecular inflammation and sarcopenia. Int J Mol Sci 2010;11(4):1509–26.
73. Marzetti E, Hwang JC, Lees HA, et al. Mitochondrial death effectors: relevance to sarcopenia and disuse muscle atrophy. Biochim Biophys Acta-General Subjects 2010;1800(3):235–44.
74. Aagaard P, Suetta C, Caserotti P, et al. Role of the nervous system in sarcopenia and muscle atrophy with aging: strength training as a countermeasure. Scand J Med Sci Sports 2010;20(1):49–64.
75. Kim JS, Wilson JM, Lee SR. Dietary implications on mechanisms of sarcopenia: roles of protein, amino acids and antioxidants. J Nutr Biochem 2010;21(1):1–13.
76. Donini LM, Chumlea WM, Vellas B, et al. Obesity in the elderly Iana symposium—Rome, 26–28th January 2006. J Nutr Health Aging 2006;10(1):52–4.
77. St-Onge MP, Gallagher D. Body composition changes with aging: The cause or the result of alterations in metabolic rate and macronutrient oxidation? Nutrition 2010;26(2):152–5.
78. Greenberg AS, Obin MS. Obesity and the role of adipose tissue in inflammation and metabolism. Am J Clin Nutr 2006;83:461S–5S.
79. Shulman GI. Cellular mechanisms of insulin resistance. J Clin Invest 2000; 106(2):171–6.
80. Chandalia M, Abate N. Metabolic complications of obesity: inflated or inflamed? J Diabetes Complications 2007;21(2):128–36.
81. Visser M, Bouter LM, McQuillan GM, et al. Elevated C-reactive protein levels in overweight and obese adults. JAMA 1999;282(22):2131–55.
82. Fried SK, Bunkin DA, Greenberg AS. Omental and subcutaneous adipose tissues of obese subjects release interleukin-6: depot difference and regulation by glucocorticoid. J Clin Endocrinol Metab 1998;83(3):847–50.
83. Weisberg SP, McCann D, Desai M, et al. Obesity is associated with macrophage accumulation in adipose tissue. J Clin Invest 2003;112(12):1796–808.
84. Roubenoff R. Sarcopenic obesity: does muscle loss cause fat gain? lessons from rheumatoid arthritis and osteoarthritis. Ann N Y Acad Sci 2005;904(1): 553–7.
85. Vandervoot AA, Symons TB. Functional and metabolic consequences of sarcopenia. Can J Appl Physiol-Revue Canadienne De Physiologie Appliquee 2001; 26(1):90–101.
86. Visser M, Goodpaster BH, Kritchevsky SB, et al. Muscle mass, muscle strength, and muscle fat infiltration as predictors of incident mobility limitations in well-functioning older persons. J Gerontol B Psychol Sci Soc Sci 2005;60(3):324–33.
87. Visser M, Newman AB, Nevitt MC, et al. Reexamining the sarcopenia hypothesis. Muscle mass versus muscle strength. Health, Aging, and Body Composition Study Research Group. Ann N Y Acad Sci 2000;904:456–61.
88. Goodpaster BH, Park SW, Harris TB, et al. The loss of skeletal muscle strength, mass, and quality in older adults: the health, aging and body composition study. J Gerontol A Biol Sci Med Sci 2006;61(10):1059–64.
89. Janssen I. Influence of sarcopenia on the development of physical disability: the Cardiovascular Health Study. J Am Geriatr Soc 2006;54(1):56–62.

90. Dey DK, Bosaeus I, Lissner L, et al. Changes in body composition and its relation to muscle strength in 75-year-old men and women: a 5-year prospective follow-up study of the NORA cohort in Goteborg, Sweden. Nutrition 2009;25(6):613–9.
91. Lee JS, Auyeung TW, Kwok T, et al. Associated factors and health impact of sarcopenia in older Chinese men and women: a cross-sectional study. Gerontology 2007;53(6):404–10.
92. Faulkner JA, Davis CS, Mendias CL, et al. The aging of elite male athletes: age-related changes in performance and skeletal muscle structure and function. Clin J Sport Med 2008;18(6):501–7.
93. Waters DL, Mullins PG, Qualls CR, et al. Mitochondrial function in physically active elders with sarcopenia. Mech Ageing Dev 2009;130(5):315–9.
94. Cosqueric G, Sebag A, Ducolombier C, et al. Sarcopenia is predictive of nosocomial infection in care of the elderly. Br J Nutr 2006;96(5):895–901.
95. Roubenoff R. Excess baggage: sarcopenia, obesity, and cancer outcomes. Lancet Oncol 2008;9(7):605–7.
96. Romero-Corral A, Somers VK, Sierra-Johnson J, et al. Accuracy of body mass index in diagnosing obesity in the adult general population. Int J Obes (Lond) 2008;32(6):959–66.
97. Alley DE, Chang VW. The changing relationship of obesity and disability, 1988–2004. JAMA 2007;298(17):2020–7.
98. Al Snih S, Ottenbacher KJ, Markides KS, et al. The effect of obesity on disability vs mortality in older Americans. Arch Intern Med 2007;167:774–80.
99. Ferrucci L, Alley D. Obesity, disability, and mortality: a puzzling link. Arch Intern Med 2007;167(8):750–1.
100. Friedmann JM, Elasy T, Jensen GL. The relationship between body mass index and self-reported functional limitation among older adults: a gender difference. J Am Geriatr Soc 2001;49(4):398–403.
101. Sternfeld B, Ngo L, Satariano WA, et al. Associations of body composition with physical performance and self-reported functional limitation in elderly men and women. Am J Epidemiol 2002;156(2):110–21.
102. Newman AB, Haggerty CL, Goodpaster B, et al. Strength and muscle quality in a well-functioning cohort of older adults: the health, aging and body composition study. J Am Geriatr Soc 2003;51(3):323–30.
103. Villareal DT, Banks M, Siener C, et al. Physical frailty and body composition in obese elderly men and women. Obes Res 2004;12(6):913–20.
104. Rolland Y, Lauwers-Cances V, Pahor M, et al. Muscle strength in obese elderly women: effect of recreational physical activity in a cross-sectional study. Am J Clin Nutr 2004;79(4):552–7.
105. Stenholm S, Alley D, Bandinelli S, et al. The effect of obesity combined with low muscle strength on decline in mobility in older persons: results from the InCHIANTI study. Int J Obes (Lond) 2009;33(6):635–44.
106. Rolland Y, Lauwers-Cances V, Cristini C, et al. Difficulties with physical function associated with obesity, sarcopenia, and sarcopenic-obesity in community-dwelling elderly women: the EPIDOS (EPIDemiologie de l'OSteoporose) Study. Am J Clin Nutr 2009;89(6):1895–900.
107. Bouchard DR, Dionne IJ, Brochu M. Sarcopenic/obesity and physical capacity in older men and women: data from the Nutrition as a Determinant of Successful Aging (NuAge)-the Quebec longitudinal Study. Obesity (Silver Spring) 2009;17(11):2082–8.
108. Baumgartner RN, Wayne SJ, Waters DL, et al. Sarcopenic obesity predicts instrumental activities of daily living disability in the elderly. Obes Res 2004;12(12):1995–2004.

109. Aubertin-Leheudre M, Lord C, Goulet EB, et al. Effect of sarcopenia on cardio-vascular disease risk factors in obese postmenopausal women. Obesity (Silver Spring) 2006;14(12):2277–83.

110. Aubertin-Leheudre M, Audet M, Goulet ED, et al. HRT provides no additional beneficial effect on sarcopenia in physically active postmenopausal women: a cross-sectional, observational study. Maturitas 2005;51(2):140–5.

111. Stephen WC, Janssen I. Sarcopenic-obesity and cardiovascular disease risk in the elderly. J Nutr Health Aging 2009;13(5):460–6.

112. Licastro F, Candore G, Lio D, et al. Innate immunity and inflammation in ageing: a key for understanding age-related diseases. Immun Ageing 2005;2:8.

113. Prado CM, Lieffers JR, McCargar LJ, et al. Prevalence and clinical implications of sarcopenic obesity in patients with solid tumours of the respiratory and gastrointestinal tracts: a population-based study. Lancet Oncol 2008;9(7): 629–35.

114. Monteiro MA, Gabriel RC, Sousa MF, et al. Temporal parameters of the foot roll-over during walking: influence of obesity and sarcopenic obesity on postmeno-pausal women. Maturitas 2010;67(2):178–85.

115. Monteiro M, Gabriel R, Aranha J, et al. Influence of obesity and sarcopenic obesity on plantar pressure of postmenopausal women. Clin Biomech (Bristol, Avon) 2010;25(5):461–7.

116. Manini TM, Clark BC. Dynapenia and Aging: an Update. J Gerontol A Biol Sci Med Sci 2011. [Epub ahead of print].

117. Moreland JD, Richardson JA, Goldsmith CH, et al. Muscle weakness and falls in older adults: a systematice review and meta-analysis. J Am Geriatr Soc 2004; 52:1121–9.

118. Jensen GL, Friedmann JM. Obesity is associated with fuctional decline in community-dwelling rural older persons. J Am Geriatr Soc 2002;50(5):918–23.

Current and Future Pharmacologic Treatment of Sarcopenia

Yves Rolland, MD, PhD[a,b,*], Graziano Onder, MD, PhD[c],
John E. Morley, MD, PhD[d,e], Sophie Gillette-Guyonet, PhD[a,b],
Gabor Abellan van Kan, MD[a,b], Bruno Vellas, MD, PhD[a,b]

KEYWORDS

• Sarcopenia • ACE • Testosterone • Growth hormone
• Creatine • Vitamin D • Leptin • Myostatin

Sarcopenia is a complex multifactorial condition that can by treated with multimodal approaches. No pharmacologic agent to prevent or treat sarcopenia has proven to be as efficacious as exercise (mainly resistance training) in combination with nutritional intervention (adequate protein and energy intake). This approach is currently the key strategy for the management of sarcopenia.[1] However, resistance training and following nutritional advice can be challenging, especially for frail, sarcopenic, elderly patients, and results remain only partial.

New pharmacologic agents could radically change the therapeutic approach to sarcopenia. It is unlikely that any drug will replace the multiple beneficial effects of nutrition and physical exercise, but new pharmacologic agents to prevent or treat sarcopenia may substantially reduce the functional decline in older people.

This article reviews the new pharmacologic agents currently being assessed for treating sarcopenia (**Table 1**). A discussion of new strategies based on nutrition (mainly essential amino acids) or physical activity is beyond the scope of this article.

[a] Inserm U1027, University of Toulouse III, Avenue Jules Guesdes, F-31073, Toulouse, France
[b] Gérontopôle of Toulouse, CHU Purpan, 170 Avenue de Casselardit, 31300 Toulouse, France
[c] Department of Gerontology and Geriatrics, Catholic University of Sacred Heart, Rome, Italy
[d] Geriatric Research, Education and Clinical Center, St Louis VA Medical Center, St Louis, MO, USA
[e] Division of Geriatrics, St Louis University School of Medicine, St Louis, MO, USA
* Corresponding author. Gérontopôle de Toulouse, Pavillon Junot, 170 Avenue de Casselardit, Hôpital La Grave-Casselardit, 31300 Toulouse, France.
E-mail address: rolland.y@chu-toulouse.fr

Clin Geriatr Med 27 (2011) 423–447
doi:10.1016/j.cger.2011.03.008
0749-0690/11/$ – see front matter © 2011 Elsevier Inc. All rights reserved.

Table 1
Current and future pharmacologic treatment of sarcopenia

| Drugs | Effect on Muscle Mass in Humans Documented in | | Safety Concerns in Humans | Availability on the Market | Indicated for the Treatment of Sarcopenia |
	Observational Studies	RCT			
Testosterone	Yes	Yes	Prostate cancer, erythrocytosis, hyperviscosity, obstructive sleep apnea, cardiovascular events	Yes	Yes,[21] in men with symptoms and signs of androgen deficiency and low serum testosterone levels
SARMs	No	Yes	Lack of steroid-related side effects, elevation of ALT/AST, hematocrit, lipid profile	No	No
Growth hormone	Yes	Yes, small sample	Arthralgias, gynecomastia, soft tissue edema, carpal tunnel syndrome, diabetes	Yes	No
Ghrelin	Yes	Yes, small sample	Mild edema, transient muscle pain, increased appetite	No	No
Growth hormone secretagogue	No	Yes	Fatigue, insomnia, increases in fasting glucose, glycosylated hemoglobin, indices of insulin resistance, transient elevation of ALT/AST	No	No
Melanocortin-4 receptor antagonists	No	No	(?)	No	No
Estrogens	Yes	Yes	Venous thromboembolism, cardiovascular disease, stroke, breast cancer	No	No

Leptin	Yes	No	(?)	No	No
Vitamin D	Yes	Yes	Vitamin D toxicity	Yes	Yes[1]
Myostatin inhibitor	Yes	Yes, small sample	(?) Reported safe and well tolerated	No	No
ACE inhibitors	Yes	Yes	Hyperkalemia, increase creatinine	Yes	No
Statins	Yes	No	Myotoxicity, rare	Yes	No
β-blockers	Yes	No	Fatigue, bradycardia	Yes	No
Vasodilator	Yes	No	Orthostatic hypotension, falls	Yes	No
Cytokine inhibitors	Yes	No	Immunosuppression	Yes	No
Polyunsaturated fatty acids	Yes	Yes small sample	Well tolerated Rare and mild	Yes	No
PPAR agonist	Yes	No	Fluid retention, weight gain	Yes	No
Creatine	No	Yes	Well tolerated Mild	Yes	Possible[1]
Bicarbonate	No	Yes	No	Yes	No
Gigko	No	No	Well tolerated Mild	Yes	No
Coenzyme Q	No	No	Well tolerated	Yes	No

Abbreviations: ACE, angiotensin II converting enzyme; ALT, alanine aminotransferase; AST, aspartate aminotransferase; PPAR, peroxisome proliferator–activated receptor; RCT, randomized controlled trial; SARMs, selective androgen receptor modulators; (?), unknown.

HORMONAL APPROACH
Testosterone

Testosterone levels gradually decline in elderly men at a rate of 1% per year. Hypogonadism occurs in approximately 20% of men older than 60 years and 50% of men older than 80 years.[2] Epidemiologic studies support a relationship between low levels of testosterone in elderly men and loss of muscle mass, strength, and function.[3,4]

Currently, supraphysiologic doses of testosterone are known to dramatically increase muscle mass and strength in young subjects performing resistance training. However, androgen deprivation therapy in elderly men with prostate cancer results in a substantial decrease in lean mass and physical activity, and an increased level of fatigue.[5] Basic research also supports the hypothesis that testosterone may prevent sarcopenia, because testosterone increases the rate of muscle protein synthesis and the number of muscle satellite cells.[6]

In hypogonadal elderly men, testosterone administration increased muscle mass, muscle strength, and decreased fat mass,[7–15] and has been reported to improve rehabilitation outcomes. However, inconclusive results are reported from studies evaluating its effectiveness on muscle strength, muscle power, and function in community-dwelling populations. Whether testosterone administration decreases the risk of falls, death, or disability is under debate. A meta-analysis performed in 2006 indicated that a moderate increase in muscle strength occurred among men participating in 11 randomized studies (with 1 study influencing the mean effect size).[16] These discrepancies may be explained by the characteristics of the recruited population. In healthy men aged 60 to 80 years with a low level of testosterone, 80 mg of testosterone during 6 months resulted in a 1.2 kg (0.7–1.7) increase in lean body mass, but no improvement in strength or function were recorded.[14] However, Srinivas-Shankar and colleagues[17] recently reported that in frail and intermediate frail older men, administration of 50 mg/d of transdermal testosterone over 6 months resulted in not only a significant increase in lean mass but also an increase in knee extensor strength and physical function. Testosterone supplementation may further increase muscle mass and function in frail older adults when combined with a nutritional supplement in undernourished older people,[18] or with physical exercise.[19] Large clinical trials on testosterone are still required to show that testosterone supplementation prevents functional decline and disability in frail elderly adults.[20]

Testosterone treatment is still controversial in patients with sarcopenia, mainly because of safety concerns. In 2010, application of testosterone gel was associated with an increased risk of cardiovascular adverse events in older men, with limitations in mobility and a high prevalence of chronic disease.[20] However, pedal edema was also reported, and this is often unrelated to heart failure in frail older persons. The current recommendations on testosterone therapy propose that men with consistent symptoms and signs of androgen deficiency, including low muscle mass and strength and unequivocally low serum testosterone levels, should be treated.[21] The potential adverse effects recommend against starting testosterone in patients with clinical or biologic suspicion of prostate cancer, erythrocytosis, hyperviscosity, untreated obstructive sleep apnea, lower urinary tract symptoms, or class III or IV heart failure.[22] Patients should be monitored and the treatment evaluated closely. Failure to relieve symptoms after a period of 4 to 6 months justifies reconsidering the treatment.[23]

Synthetic androgen modulators, such as the 7 α-methyl-19-nortesterone (ie, MENT or trestolone) or selective androgen receptor modulators (SARMs), are potential alternatives to testosterone. SARMs have the same anabolic effects on muscle tissue as testosterone in rodents but without the undesirable side effects, such as virilizing effects.[24] A single trial in healthy older men and women showed that the SARM ostarine increased muscle mass and stair climbing power after 3 months.[25] These drugs may expand the clinical application of androgen modulators in sarcopenic men and women as they enter the clinical phase of research.[26]

Growth Hormone, Growth Hormone Secretagogue, and Ghrelin

Growth hormone (GH) promotes muscle growth through favoring the maturation of muscle satellites cells. It also induces an increase in muscular oxidative enzymes and fatigue resistance through improving muscle mitochondrial functioning. These effects are mediated by insulin-like growth factor I (IGF-1) produced by the liver or locally produced by muscle in response to GH or exercise. IGF-1 also downregulates the production proinflammatory cytokines. GH level declines at a rate of 1% per year after 30 years of age. Approximately 30% of older men older than 60 years have been found to be GH-deficient.[27] However, conflicting results have been reported during GH supplementation in older people with somatopause.

In older men, numerous clinical trial have failed to show any additional benefit of GH supplementation combined with exercise training or other anabolic hormones on muscle fiber hypertrophy, muscle strength, muscle power, or IGF-1 expression.[28–31] These negative results may be explained by the absence of the physiologic pulsatile pattern during exogenous GH supplementation and the GH-related insulin resistance, but also by methodological issues such as the small sample size of most trials. Moreover, in most of the studies a high incidence of side effects were reported, including arthralgias, gynecomastia, soft tissue edema, carpal tunnel syndrome, and diabetes, and resulted in numerous treatment withdrawals. These results raise serious concerns in clinical practice.

In a clinical trial among obese postmenopausal women, the administration of GH alone or in combination with IGF-I resulted in a greater reduction of weight and fat mass than was achieved with diet and exercise alone, without compromising fat-free mass.[32] However, another small clinical trial found no clear additional effect when combining GH and IGF-1 in older people.[33]

However, other studies reported that a few months of GH supplementation significantly increased lower-extremity muscle strength and muscle mass in healthy older men and women[34] and women with osteoporosis.[35]

In 2009, Sattler and colleagues[36] also reported on a group of older men and found that those who received the highest doses of combined supplementation of GH (5 μg/kg per day) with testosterone (10 g/d) for 4 months increased their lean mass by a mean 3 kg (maximum increase of 7.5 kg) and their muscle strength by 30%. During the same period, the mean fat mass decreased by 2.3 kg (maximum decrease of 7.1 kg).

Previously, one study performed in 10 older men found no change in lean mass or strength after 1 month of 6.25 μg/kg per day of recombinant human GH combined with 5 mg/d of testosterone,[37] whereas another trial involving 74 older men who received 20 to 30 μg/kg of recombinant human GH three times per week plus 100 mg of intramuscular testosterone two times a week for 26 weeks showed a 4.3-kg increase in lean mass, compared with 3.1 kg in those treated with testosterone alone.[38] No clinically relevant improvement in muscle performance was seen in these studies.

Ghrelin is a peptide hormone produced by the stomach in response to fasting. An increase in ghrelin blood concentration results in an elevated sensation of hunger and increased food intake. This effect is partly related to melanocortin receptor antagonism, which modulates food intake. Ghrelin inhibits the central melanocortin system involved in the pathogenesis of cachexia in rats.[39] This effect has led researchers to explore ghrelin (or ghrelin agonist) as a potential therapy for reducing wasting in chronic diseases and cachexia, with promising effects recently reported.[40,41] In 25 cachectic patients with chronic obstructive pulmonary disorder, subcutaneous injections of a synthetic ghrelin analog tended to increase lean mass and physical performances with no added safety issues.[41]

Apart from other activities, ghrelin also stimulates the release of GH through activation of the GH secretagogue-receptor 1a (GHS-R 1a) present in the hypothalamus, and ghrelin mimetic restores the pulsatile GH secretion in older adults. Therefore, GH secretagogue or GH secretagogue–receptor agonist may modulate muscle mass in older adults. Ghrelin concentrations have been reported to be strongly related to the amount of skeletal muscle mass.[42] Very few clinical trials on synthetic ghrelin or ghrelin agonist therapy have been published in older people. In healthy older adults without sarcopenia, 2 years of an oral ghrelin mimetic increased GH and IGF-1 blood levels and fat-free mass (1.1 kg [0.7–1.5 kg] vs −0.5 kg [−1.1–0.2 kg] for the placebo group) but produced no significant changes in strength or function.[43] The treatment was well tolerated. In healthy volunteers, oral ghrelin mimetic was shown to increase body mass[44] after 1 week. At 6 months, administration of capromorelin, a GH secretagogue, increased lean body mass by 1.4 kg (0.3 kg in the placebo group) but also significantly improved the physical performances of older adults.[45]

Melanocortin-4 Receptor Antagonists

The central melanocortin system seems important in the pathogenesis of cachexia. Its effect on feeding behavior and the metabolic rate is mediated by the melanocortin-4 receptor (MC4R) that is predominantly present in the brain. Stimulation of the MC4R results in anorexia, weight loss, and increased metabolic rate. In humans, mutations of the MC4R resulted in severe obesity.[46] However, blockade of central melanocortin signaling increased both lean body mass and fat mass in a rat model of cardiac cachexia.[47]

Several studies on new treatment approaches to cachexia have been presented recently. A MC4R antagonist was reported to have beneficial effect in attenuating body composition changes related to cachexia.[41,48] Clinical trials in humans should be reported soon.

Estrogens and Tibolone

Women experience an accelerated loss of muscle mass and strength around the time of menopause.[49,50] Changes in lifestyle habits, such as low level of physical activity during this period, and hormonal changes may be the two main determinants of loss of muscle mass and strength. Evidence linking hormonal replacement therapy and muscle mass and strength has been reported. However, controversy still exists regarding the role of estrogen or tibolone, a synthetic steroid with oestrogenic, progestagenic, and androgenic activity, on skeletal muscle in postmenopausal women. Very few clinical trials on estrogens and tibolone included older women.[15]

Among the five clinical trials that have assessed the effect of estrogens on muscle strength, three reported a statistically significant improvement of muscle strength while the two others were negative.[51] The effect of estrogen on muscle mass is also controversial, with some studies suggesting that estrogen can increase lean body mass or decrease fat mass, and other studies showing no effects.[15] Moreover, the risk–benefit balance of the estrogen therapy must be incorporated into the discussion.[52]

However, tibolone showed a significant positive effect on muscle strength (evidenced only in one clinical trial)[53] and a significant effect on muscle mass in most studies published.[54–58] The functional benefit of tibolone may also be related to its positive effect on fat mass.[51,56] Improvement of quality of life in postmenopausal women undergoing hormonal replacement therapy may also be related to a significant reduction of symptoms, such as aching muscles.[59]

Estrogen and tibolone may both react with intranuclear receptors in muscle fibers,[60,61] and tibolone may also bind androgen receptors in muscle fibers and increase free testosterone and GH. In postmenopausal women, estrogen replacement therapy results in a higher myogenic regulatory factor gene expression, a greater myogenic response to maximal eccentric exercise,[62] and a reduced muscle damage after maximal eccentric exercise.[63] Furthermore, estrogen replacement therapy has been reported to improve insulin response during an exercise training.[64] Insulin's role in the origin and pathogenesis of sarcopenia is important.

Currently, evidence of a muscle effect of estrogen is shown in a few short-term clinical trials performed in small samples of postmenopausal women and very few in older people. The long-term safety and side effects must be addressed in this indication.

Leptin

Leptin is an adipokine secreted by the adipose tissue that downregulates satiety and the size of adipose tissue mass.[65] Leptin has also been reported to regulate several physiologic processes, including skeletal muscle protein synthesis.[66] The role of leptin on sarcopenia is poorly understood, however. Leptin-deficient mice are obese and display a reduced skeletal muscle mass.[67] In these leptin-deficient ob/ob mice, muscle mass increased with leptin administration.[68] Moreover, leptin administration is associated with an inactivation of several atrogenes (Fox, MAFbx, and MuRF1, which are markers of muscle atrophy), a decrease in myostatin, and an increase in peroxisome proliferator–activated receptor-γ coactivator-1α (PGC-1α).[68] Whether these changes are related to hormonal changes, such as in testosterone or GH levels; leptin administration; or changes in physical activity requires further investigation.

In clinical practice, obese patients may not be the target population to benefit from leptin therapy because they exhibit hyperleptinemia and leptin resistance, and usually have more muscle mass than patients who are not obese. This leptin resistance seems to be caused by hypertriglyceridemia, and therefore lowering triglycerides may overcome the leptin resistance.[69] However, leptin may be a promising approach to prevent muscle loss during bed rest, limb disuse, or cachexia.

Vitamin D

The current nutritional recommendations for the management of sarcopenia are to measure levels of 25(OH) vitamin D in all patients with sarcopenia and to provide a supplement for all with a value less than 100 nmol/L.[1] Proximal muscle weakness is a usual clinical symptom of vitamin D deficiency. Prevalence of a low level of vitamin D has been repeatedly reported to be high in older people, and is still significant in the older population.[70–72]

Vitamin D has the potential to improve muscle strength. A longitudinal epidemiologic study reported an independent association between low serum vitamin D and the loss of muscle strength and muscle mass.[73] Randomized controlled trials reported that vitamin D supplementation increased muscle strength.[74–76] Several randomized controlled trials in adults aged 65 years and older have also reported that 800 IU of vitamin D_3 significantly improved lower-extremity strength and function by 4% to 11%[74,75,77] and body sway by 28%[75,77] after 2 to 12 months.

As a result, vitamin D can also reduce the risk for falls and fractures.[78] A recent meta-analysis reported that 700 to 1000 IU/d of vitamin D reduces the risk of falling by 19% in older people.[79]

The reduction in the risk for falls is at least partly related to the direct effect of vitamin D on muscle tissue. Muscle anabolism decreases when vitamin D level is low.[80] Low vitamin D levels also influence muscle protein turnover through reduced insulin secretion and increased myofibrillar degradation.[81] Janssen and colleagues[82] reported histologic muscle atrophy, predominantly type II fibers, in vitamin D deficiency, and an increase in the number and size of type II muscle fibers after 3 months of treatment with 1-alpha-calcidiol in postmenopausal women with osteoporosis.[83] Membrane and nuclear receptors have been described in muscle cells in human.[84,85] Nuclear 1,25 hydroxyvitamin D receptors are members of the steroid hormone superfamily. These receptors have various genetic polymorphisms, which have been associated with fat-free mass.[86] 1,25 hydroxyvitamin D and 1,25 hydroxyvitamin D receptors have a direct effect on both the metabolic processes and the transcriptional regulation of skeletal muscle.[87] In combination with cofactors, vitamin D linked with its nuclear receptor can modulate gene expression of proteins, such as those involved the metabolism of calcium or IGF binding protein-3.[87] Muscle function may also be influenced by 1,25 hydroxyvitamin D membrane receptors through their ability to modulate the membrane calcium channels of the muscle fibers.[88] This effect is rapid and seems independent of the intranuclear transcription process.

Myostatin

Myostatin is a member of the transforming growth factor-β (TGF-β) family, which is expressed in skeletal muscle, and inhibits muscle growth.[89] Myostatin downregulates the Akt/mammalian target of rapamycin (Akt/mTOR) pathway. Myostatin decreases protein synthesis and muscle cell synthesis.[90] Myostatin represents an important potential therapeutic approach for sarcopenia and other muscular disorders, such as muscular dystrophy.

In animals and humans, mutations in the myostatin gene result in increased muscle mass.[91,92] A single gene administration of myostatin inhibitor enhances muscle mass and strength in mouse.[93] Antagonism of myostatin enhanced muscle tissue regeneration in aged mice.[92] The increase in muscle mass is caused by both hypertrophy and hyperplasia.[94]

Different approaches to inhibit the effect of myostatin are currently in development.[95] Hormones such as follistatin, a myostatin-binding protein, and drugs such as trichostatin A can antagonize myostatin and are potential new therapeutic for patients with sarcopenia.[96–99] The effects of follistatin, originally named follicle-stimulating hormone (FSH)–suppressing protein, are multiple. It induces muscle hypertrophy through satellite cell proliferation by inhibiting both myostatin and activin.[100]

Activin is another TGF-β expressed by the muscle. At the 5th Cachexia Conference held in December 2009 in Barcelona, Spain, Kate Murphy from the University of Melbourne, Australia, presented on the effects of myostatin antibody on skeletal muscle in aged mice.[41] The authors reported a statistically significant increased muscle mass by 8% to 18%, muscle fiber size by 12%, and muscle strength by 35% after 14 weeks of treatment. At the same time, percentage of type IIa fibers increased by 114% and muscle fiber oxidative capacity improved by 39%.[41] Recombinant human antibodies to myostatin are currently being tested in humans with muscular dystrophy.

The other approach is to use a soluble myostatin decoy receptor (activin type IIB receptor; ActRIIB-Fc) or an extracellular domain of the human ActRIIB receptor. In the Barcelona meeting, Peter Bialek from Pfizer in Cambridge, Massachusetts, reported on cachexia models of mice, showing promising results of ActRIIB-Fc on muscle mass and function.[41] In a randomized, double-blind, phase I study in healthy postmenopausal women, Jasbir Seehra from Acceleron Pharma in Cambridge, Massachusetts, reported a 2.4% to 2.6% increase in lean body mass after only 15 days of treatment. The treatment was safe and well tolerated.[41] In the future, gene administration of myostatin inhibitor proteins may also be a option to enhance muscle mass and strength.[93] However, experts have reported that muscle tissue may be more susceptible to muscle and tendon injuries in mice with myostatin deficiency.[101]

CARDIOVASCULAR DRUGS ANGIOTENSIN II-CONVERTING ENZYME INHIBITORS

Angiotensin II-converting enzyme (ACE) inhibitors improve the vital prognostic of patients with congestive heart failure, and can also reduce their functional decline. This beneficial effect is attributable to the cardiovascular actions but may also be related to the direct effect of ACE inhibitors on the skeletal muscle tissue.[15,102–105] The activation of the renin-angiotensin-aldosterone system may be involved in the progress of sarcopenia, and growing evidence from basic and clinical research suggests that ACE inhibitors may prevent sarcopenia.[106]

In the Health, Aging and Body Composition (Health ABC) study, a cross-sectional association of the ACE inhibitor users with lower-extremity lean body mass was reported, even after adjustment for potential confounders.[107] This association was not reported with the other antihypertensive drugs. Among the 641 participants of the observational Women's Health and Aging Study, Onder and colleagues[106] reported a lower rate of lower-extremity muscle strength and walking speed decline at 3 years in the ACE inhibitor users than in continuous or intermittent users of other antihypertensive drugs.

The effect of the ACE inhibitor on physical function in elderly people with functional impairment was examined in only three previous randomized controlled trials. In the Trial of Angiotensin-Converting Enzyme Inhibition and Novel Cardiovascular Risk Factors (TRAIN) study, no beneficial effect on physical performances was reported in the older subjects randomized during 6 months in the ACE inhibitors group compared with the placebo group.[108] In the second study, physical performances of hypertensive elderly subjects randomized to either ACE inhibitors or calcium inhibitor during 9 months were similar.[109] Previously, Sumukadas and colleagues[110] reported promising results. In this third study, 130 elderly participants with no heart failure or left ventricular systolic dysfunction were enrolled. Over 20 weeks of treatment, the 6-minute walking distance was significantly improved in the ACE inhibitor group relative to the placebo group, with a mean between-group difference of 31.4 m. This effect was similar to the improvement expected with exercise training.

ACE inhibitors have been reported to be involved in various extracardiovascular mechanisms, including those involving muscle tissue. The ACE gene polymorphism affects the muscle anabolic response and muscular efficiency after physical training.[104] A lower ACE activity has been reported in carriers of the I allele (for insertion of a 287-bp fragment) , whereas a higher ACE activity is found in carriers of the D allele (for deletion).[111] However, conflicted results have been reported on the effect of this deletion/insertion polymorphism. A Danish epidemiologic study reported no substantial effects of ACE genotype on physical performance among older adults.[112] However, another cohort showed that carriers of the ACE II allele gene polymorphism had improved endurance capability,[113] and also had a greater anabolic response to an exercise training program. Among athletes, the ACE II allele polymorphism seems to be associated with a higher percentage of type I (slow twitch) than of type II (fast twitch) muscle fibers,[114] and power performance.[115] The mechanical efficiency of human muscle has also been shown to increase in response to training in carriers of the II allele.[116] Subjects with the homozygous DD allele showed greater strength enhancement in response to resistance exercise training.[117] This genotype is associated with a risk of developing hypertension cardiac related to the smooth muscle hypertrophy, but it may also induce skeletal muscle hypertrophy (specifically of the type II fast-twitch fibers) after resistance training. Some authors suggest an increased skeletal muscle quality (force output/muscle mass) but not an absolute increase of skeletal muscle quantity in carriers of the DD allele.[118]

The biologic mechanisms involved in the greater improvement in muscle efficiency reported after endurance training in subjects with low ACE activity is not clearly elucidated. Endurance training can result in quantitative and qualitative changes in muscle tissue, such as the efficiency of mitochondrial respiration, the development of muscle capillary network, or transition in isoforms of myosin heavy chain. The direct effects of ACE activity on myosin heavy chain expression remain controversial.

Recent findings suggest that the improvement of functional response to endurance training with an ACE inhibitor is not explained by changes in muscle oxidative capacity or contractile phenotype[119] but rather by peripheral oxygenation. Increased muscle capillary bed could explain the enhancement of muscle efficiency. A reduction in microvessel density and of insulin signaling occurs in the skeletal muscle tissue of untreated hypertensive rats that can be restored by angiotensin receptor blockers.[120] ACE inhibitors increase capillary density of skeletal muscle in response to exercise,[121] and may also produce a lower formation of angiotensin II and an increased formation of bradykinin during endurance training, and thus an improved vasodilatation. Oxygen and substrate delivery to the skeletal muscles tissue would be improved. In the ischemic limb of normotensive and hypertensive animals, ACE inhibitors increase angiogenesis and collateral vessel growth.[122] Moreover, ACE inhibitor improve insulin sensitivity[123] and restore the impaired insulin-mediated capillary recruitment in skeletal muscle during diabetes.[124]

The renin-angiotensin system mediates the inflammatory response, an important factor in the development of sarcopenia. Activation of the renin-angiotensin system results in increased proinflammatory cytokine production[125] and therefore promotes the degradation of muscle proteins. Angiotensin II infused in rats resulted in muscle atrophy.[96] In patients with cachexia, those with the D allele (higher ACE activity) showed lower lean body mass than those with the II allele.[118] In human vascular smooth muscle cells, angiotensin II induces IL-6 release[126] and stimulates matrix metalloproteinase secretion through activation of nuclear factor-kappa B.[127] These mechanisms can be reversed by ACE inhibitors in vitro and in vivo. This decrease in inflammatory markers via ACE inhibitors may also improve microvascular endothelial function and blood flow, consequently slowing muscle loss.[128] Brull and colleagues[129] reported that subjects treated with ACE inhibitors after coronary artery bypass surgery had a significantly lower increase in IL-6 concentration compared with nontreated participants. Angiotensin II receptor antagonists attenuate the cytokine production. This effect may be related to the activation of peroxisome proliferator–activated receptor (PPAR) γ, which has an anti-inflammatory effect.[130] These effects have been reported in vascular smooth muscle cells, but angiotensin II receptor antagonist was shown to attenuate hepatic inflammation in animals[131] and may also be involved in skeletal tissue. In skeletal muscle tissue, angiotensin II receptor blocker improved skeletal muscle fatty acid oxidation through a modulation of PPAR-γ and may have an important role in the regulation of muscle bioenergetics.[132]

The GH/IGF-1 axis is modulated by the ACE inhibitors.[133] IGF-1 is a potential contributor to sarcopenia. It activates satellite cell proliferation and differentiation, and increases protein synthesis in existing fibers.[134] ACE inhibitors may prevent the loss of muscle mass through modulation of the IGF-1 system. This effect may be related to the reduction of the autocrine IGF-1 system.[96,135] In the SIRENTE study,[136] or the InCHIANTI study,[137] ACE inhibitor use by older adults was associated with higher levels of IGF-binding protein-3.

The direct effect of ACE inhibitors on the IGF-1 system has been reported in different large epidemiologic cohorts of older people.[136,137] However, overexpression of the muscle-specific isoform of IGF-1 mitigates angiotensin II-induced muscle loss.[133] Other hormones may be involved. Protein synthesis in response to insulin seems to be impaired in the aging muscle cell, and ACE inhibition associated with the I allele increases insulin sensitivity, reflected by higher glucose uptake and glycogen stores in skeletal muscle.[117] Skeletal muscle capillary increases to augment glucose delivery during physiologic hyperinsulinemia. In Zucker obese diabetic rats, ACE-I therapy was reported to improve this insulin-mediated capillary recruitment in skeletal muscle.[124]

Statins

A large number of clinical trials have shown that statins reduce major cardiovascular events, but they have also been recognized to cause occasional adverse effects on skeletal muscle mass.[138] Statins may reduce aerobic exercise tolerance through impaired mitochondrial function, decreased mitochondrial content, and apoptotic pathways.[139] In a longitudinal study performed in community-dwelling older adults, statin therapy was associated with greater declines in strength and tended to increase the risk of falls,[140] whereas other authors reported no evidence that statin use leads to muscle strength declines[141] or modest improvement in the timed chair stand test.[142] In more than 25 000 women older than 65 years, statin use was not associated with the development of frailty as defined by the Rand-36 physical function scale.[143]

However, a significant increased appendicular lean mass was observed in statin users in several longitudinal studies,[140] especially after resistance training.[144] Several hypotheses have been reported. Statin therapy may result in small muscle tissue injuries, increase local level of growth factors, and finally cause muscle hypertrophy. Muscle perfusion and inflammation are important contributors to sarcopenia that may be modulated by statins.[15] However, statin has been reported not to improve muscle microvascular function in obese adults despite decreased inflammation.[145] These results may also be related to the limited ability of dual X-ray absorptiometry to distinguish fat tissue infiltration within muscle from muscle tissue.

Future studies are required to determine the effect of statins on skeletal muscle strength, endurance, and aerobic exercise performance.[146]

β-Blockers

β-Blockers decrease endurance exercise capacity through reducing cardiac rate and contractility via the β1 receptor. Improvement of endurance capacity during aerobic training is substantially attenuated with β-blockers, mainly when the β-blockers used are nonselective.[147] Skeletal muscle tissue expresses predominantly β2 receptors, and nonselective β-blockers may also decrease endurance exercise capacity through interactions with the skeletal muscle mitochondrial adaptations to training. PGC-1α is a transcription coactivator that increases after exercise, promotes mitochondrial biogenesis, and regulates muscle fiber type. The use of selective β1-blockers instead of nonselective β-blockers may reduce the aerobic training effects of β-blockers. β-blockers and mainly β2-blockers can reduce mitochondrial biogenesis through inhibiting the postexercise PGC-1α response.[139]

However, β-blockers may also have a beneficial effect on body weight and cachexia. β-Blockers decrease resting energy expenditure, inhibit the catecholamine-induced lipolysis,[148] and induce vasodilation of vascular smooth muscle cells via β2-receptors. In cachectic models of rats, β-blockers have been reported to reduce weight loss and improve physical activity, food intake, and survival.[41] β-Blockers may also have a positive impact on muscle protein oxidation, apoptosis, and cytokine-induced muscle loss, especially those with nitric oxide donor activity.[149]

Vasodilator

Muscle tissue perfusion contributes to the muscle protein metabolism. Vasodilatation enhances blood flow and microvascular perfusion of the muscle and is now reported to be an important contributor of muscle anabolism. Vasodilatation of skeletal muscle arterioles occurs partly through nitric oxide signaling. Insulin is also able to induce a nitric oxide–dependent vasodilation of the skeletal muscle vessels and to increase muscle perfusion.[150,151] Compared with young subjects, the muscle protein anabolic effect of insulin and the physiologic insulin-mediated nitric oxide–dependent vasodilation is decreased in older people but can be restored with vasodiltators[152–154] or exercise training.[155] During hyperinsulinemia of older adults, drugs able to restore the nitric oxide–dependent vasodilation of the muscle could restore the anabolic response of the muscle tissue to insulin.[152] However, the effect of vasodilatory drugs on muscle protein anabolism requires further investigations in humans.

ANTI-INFLAMMATORY DRUGS
Cytokine Inhibitors

The age-related inflammation process is supposed to play a crucial role in the development of sarcopenia through increasing myofibrillar protein degradation and decreasing protein synthesis. Anti-inflammatory drugs may delay its onset and progression. New drugs are currently being tested, mainly in the context of cachexia. Cytokine inhibitors, such as thalidomide, increase weight and lean tissue anabolism in patients with AIDS.[156] In a model of cardiac cachexia, anti-TNF treatment attenuated the loss of skeletal muscle mass.[157] TNF-α antibodies, a treatment provided to patients with rheumatoid arthritis, may also be an alternative therapeutic opportunity for sarcopenia.[158] Drugs that antagonize the IL-6 cytokine are currently being tested with promising results in patients with cancer complicated by severe cachexia.[41] However, the benefit/risk balance of these drugs will have to be addressed. These new approaches have currently not been tested in patients with sarcopenia.

Polyunsaturated Fatty Acids

Epidemiologic evidence suggests that polyunsaturated fatty acids (PUFAs) may prevent various impairments associated with aging, including sarcopenia. PUFAs may interfere with mechanisms (such as inflammation or oxidative damage) that contribute to loss of muscle mass.

In animals, PUFAs are known to improve aerobic capacity[159] and may improve muscle performance through inducing changes in fluidity and permeability of the membrane cell.[160] PUFAs improve muscle cell membranes in terms of fatty acid composition and are likely to facilitate insulin action.[161] In the migrating shorebird, PUFA has been reported to be a natural doping agent through improving muscle metabolism before extreme long-distance exercise.[162]

In humans, randomized controlled trials in patients with pancreatic cancer[163] or chronic obstructive pulmonary disease[164] have reported that PUFA supplementation improved exercise capacity. In a recent large epidemiologic study, the most important association between diet and grip strength was shown to occur with fatty fish consumption, a rich source of omega-3 fatty acids.[165] Others have reported conflicting epidemiologic results.[166] These findings suggest that the anti-inflammatory actions of PUFAs could prevent the mechanism leading to sarcopenia.[167] Recently, omega-3 fatty acid supplementation was reported to increase muscle protein synthesis in a small-sample randomized controlled trial of older people.[168] Whether omega-3 fatty acids are useful in preventing and treating sarcopenia must be assessed in large clinical trials.

Other Anti-Inflammatory Drugs

Other drugs can modulate the inflammatory process, such as the PPAR-δ agonist. The PPAR-δ agonist can attenuate the inflammatory process induced by fatty acids and improve insulin sensivity.[169] Cyclooxygenase inhibitors were also recently reported in older adults to improve muscle mass, muscle strength, and protein turnover in combination with resistance training programs.[170] Further research is needed to confirm these results.

METABOLIC AGENTS
Creatine

Creatine supplementation increases energy storage through increasing intramuscular phosphocreatin.[171] It may enable increased physical working capacity and resistance training, which stimulate muscle mass synthesis.[172] The benefit of creatine on exercise performances has been reported repeatedly in young adults, and creatine was recently proposed to be a potential medication for the prevention and management of sarcopenia.[1] However, few clinical trials in older people of creatine supplementation (in addition to physical training or not) report conflicting results. Some have reported that creatine increases lean mass by 1.7 kg[171] to 3.3 kg[173] after 12 to 14 weeks of resistance training, whereas others failed to observe an increase in lean mass.[174–177] In a small sample trial, creatine supplementation over 14 days improved grip strength, but no improvement in the physical performances score was noted.[178] Another study performed over 21 days in 30 women aged 58 to 71 years reported an improvement in both strength and physical performance after 7 days of creatine supplementation.[172] Other studies have reported an improvement of muscle strength and mass with creatine supplementation combined with linoleic acid and resistance training,[179,180] or in addition to protein supplementation.[181] These findings support an interactive effect between creatine and other compounds, and that coingestion of creatine with linoleic acid or amino acid may be relevant. Long-term clinical trials on the effect of creatine on muscle mass, muscle strength, and physical performances are warranted.

The rationale of creatine use relies on several biologic hypotheses. Creatine may both decrease the rate of protein catabolism and increase the rate of protein synthesis.[182] In young adults, creatine supplementation was reported to reduce whole-body protein breakdown.[183] Creatine may reduce the oxidant stress through scavenging reactive oxygen and nitrogen species.[184] It may also increase muscle mass and strength through modulating specific muscle genes, such as myogenin and muscle regulatory factor 4 (MRF-4).[185] In young adults, creatine supplementation in combination with resistance training increased mRNA and protein expression of myogenin and MRF-4.[186] Protein synthesis may also be promoted by creatine-induced intracellular water retention. Recently, creatine supplementation in combination with strength training was reported to enhance satellite cell activation and total myonuclei number per muscle fiber in young adults.[187]

Other Metabolic Agents (Bicarbonate, Gigko biloba, Coenzyme Q)

Several new pharmacologic approaches to sarcopenia have been recently suggested. These proposals are appealing because they rely on safe and well-tolerated drugs that could be prescribed in the long-term. In a double-blind, randomized, controlled trial, Dawson-Hughes and colleagues[188] explored the muscle performance of 163 healthy older adults assigned to receive either 67.5 mmol of bicarbonate or placebo. After 3 months, the mean lower-extremity muscle performance of women in the bicarbonate group significantly improved by approximately 10% relative to those in the placebo group. Grip strength also improved, but the difference between groups was not statistically significant.

The standardized Ginkgo biloba extract EGb 761 has been reported to delay the progress of sarcopenia in *Caenorhabditis elegans*.[189] In aged rats, Ginkgo biloba induced an increase in muscular mass and performance and improved muscle protein metabolism,[190] but basic research is scare and no data are currently available in humans.

Finally, nutritional mixtures, such as the Q-ter that contains terclatrated coenzyme Q10 (CoQ10); creatine; and ginseng extract have been reported to preserve physical performance in old rats. CoQ10 is a component of the electron transport chain and plays a key role in mitochondrial bioenergetics. The efficacy was, however, variable according to the age at which supplementation was provided, and was not effective in the oldest rats.[191] Moreover, other authors have reported that prolonged intake of CoQ10 impairs cognitive functions in mice.[192]

SUMMARY

Sarcopenia is a major cause of frailty and disability in older persons.[193,194] Relevant new pharmacologic drugs for sarcopenia will have a dramatic impact on improving the health and quality of life for elderly patients, reducing the associated comorbidity and disability and stabilizing rising health care costs. However, further clinical research on their effects on muscle physiology is needed before these new rising therapeutic can be recommended. The long-term safety and side effects must be taken into consideration in this frail population. Specific pharmacologic approaches may have theoretical benefits on muscle physiologic pathways but may also have deleterious effects on other organs. New therapeutic approaches to sarcopenia and its relation to the functional decline in elderly is just beginning to be studied. For example, more than 2200 randomized controlled trials are registered in Pubmed.gov with the keyword *osteoporosis*, another relevant condition related to body composition changes, whereas only 43 randomized controlled trials have been published with the keyword *sarcopenia*. The new drugs being studied will have to show their efficacy on physical performance outcomes in addition to muscle mass and strength, and target populations will have to be defined. As of 2010, vitamin D is the safest and simplest therapeutic agent that should be supplemented in all patients with sarcopenia and a low blood level of vitamin D.[1] However, in the near future patients with sarcopenia will probably benefit from a larger panel of treatments.

REFERENCES

1. Morley JE, Argiles JM, Evans WJ, et al. Nutritional recommendations for the management of sarcopenia. J Am Med Dir Assoc 2009;11(6):391–6.
2. Morley JE, Kaiser FE, Perry HM III, et al. Longitudinal changes in testosterone, luteinizing hormone, and follicle-stimulating hormone in healthy older men. Metabolism 1997;46(4):410–3.
3. Baumgartner RN, Waters DL, Gallagher D, et al. Predictors of skeletal muscle mass in elderly men and women. Mech Ageing Dev 1999;107(2):123–36.
4. Perry HM, Miller DK, Patrick P, et al. Testosterone and leptin in older African-American men: relationship to age, strength, function, and season. Metabolism 2000;49(8):1085–91.
5. Galvao DA, Spry NA, Taaffe DR, et al. Changes in muscle, fat and bone mass after 36 weeks of maximal androgen blockade for prostate cancer. BJU Int 2008;102(1):44–7.
6. Rolland Y, Czerwinski S, Abellan Van Kan G, et al. Sarcopenia: its assessment, etiology, pathogenesis, consequences and future perspectives. J Nutr Health Aging 2008;12(7):433–50.
7. Tenover JS. Effects of testosterone supplementation in the aging male. J Clin Endocrinol Metab 1992;75(4):1092–8.
8. Morley JE, Perry HM III, Kaiser FE, et al. Effects of testosterone replacement therapy in old hypogonadal males: a preliminary study. J Am Geriatr Soc 1993;41(2):149–52.
9. Katznelson L, Finkelstein JS, Schoenfeld DA, et al. Increase in bone density and lean body mass during testosterone administration in men with acquired hypogonadism. J Clin Endocrinol Metab 1996;81(12):4358–65.
10. Sih R, Morley JE, Kaiser FE, et al. Testosterone replacement in older hypogonadal men: a 12-month randomized controlled trial. J Clin Endocrinol Metab 1997; 82(6):1661–7.
11. Ly LP, Jimenez M, Zhuang TN, et al. A double-blind, placebo-controlled, randomized clinical trial of transdermal dihydrotestosterone gel on muscular strength, mobility, and quality of life in older men with partial androgen deficiency. J Clin Endocrinol Metab 2001;86(9):4078–88.
12. Kenny AM, Prestwood KM, Gruman CA, et al. Effects of transdermal testosterone on bone and muscle in older men with low bioavailable testosterone levels. J Gerontol A Biol Sci Med Sci 2001;56(5):M266–72.
13. Wittert GA, Chapman IM, Haren MT, et al. Oral testosterone supplementation increases muscle and decreases fat mass in healthy elderly males with low-normal gonadal status. J Gerontol A Biol Sci Med Sci 2003;58(7): 618–25.
14. Emmelot-Vonk MH, Verhaar HJ, Nakhai Pour HR, et al. Effect of testosterone supplementation on functional mobility, cognition, and other parameters in older men: a randomized controlled trial. JAMA 2008;299(1):39–52.
15. Onder G, Della Vedova C, Landi F. Validated treatments and therapeutics prospectives regarding pharmacological products for sarcopenia. J Nutr Health Aging 2009;13(8):746–56.
16. Ottenbacher KJ, Ottenbacher ME, Ottenbacher AJ, et al. Androgen treatment and muscle strength in elderly men: a meta-analysis. J Am Geriatr Soc 2006; 54(11):1666–73.
17. Srinivas-Shankar U, Roberts SA, Connolly MJ, et al. Effects of testosterone on muscle strength, physical function, body composition, and quality of life in

intermediate-frail and frail elderly men: a randomized, double-blind, placebo-controlled study. J Clin Endocrinol Metab 2010;95(2):639–50.

18. Chapman IM, Visvanathan R, Hammond AJ, et al. Effect of testosterone and a nutritional supplement, alone and in combination, on hospital admissions in undernourished older men and women. Am J Clin Nutr 2009;89(3):880–9.

19. Kenny AM, Boxer RS, Kleppinger A, et al. Dehydroepiandrosterone combined with exercise improves muscle strength and physical function in frail older women. J Am Geriatr Soc 2010;58(9):1707–14.

20. Basaria S, Coviello AD, Travison TG, et al. Adverse events associated with testosterone administration. N Engl J Med 2010;363(2):109–22.

21. Wang C, Nieschlag E, Swerdloff R, et al. Investigation, treatment, and monitoring of late-onset hypogonadism in males: ISA, ISSAM, EAU, EAA, and ASA recommendations. J Androl 2009;30(1):1–9.

22. Bhasin S, Cunningham GR, Hayes FJ, et al. Testosterone therapy in adult men with androgen deficiency syndromes: an endocrine society clinical practice guideline. J Clin Endocrinol Metab 2006;91(6):1995–2010.

23. Bain J. Testosterone and the aging male: to treat or not to treat? Maturitas 2010; 66(1):16–22.

24. Li JJ, Sutton JC, Nirschl A, et al. Discovery of potent and muscle selective androgen receptor modulators through scaffold modifications. J Med Chem 2007;50(13):3015–25.

25. Morley JE. Developing novel therapeutic approaches to frailty. Curr Pharm Des 2009;15(29):3384–95.

26. Gao W, Dalton JT. Expanding the therapeutic use of androgens via selective androgen receptor modulators (SARMs). Drug Discov Today 2007;12(5–6): 241–8.

27. Rudman D, Kutner MH, Rogers CM, et al. Impaired growth hormone secretion in the adult population: relation to age and adiposity. J Clin Invest 1981;67(5): 1361–9.

28. Taaffe DR, Pruitt L, Reim J, et al. Effect of recombinant human growth hormone on the muscle strength response to resistance exercise in elderly men. J Clin Endocrinol Metab 1994;79(5):1361–6.

29. Yarasheski KE, Zachwieja JJ, Campbell JA, et al. Effect of growth hormone and resistance exercise on muscle growth and strength in older men. Am J Physiol 1995;268(2 Pt 1):E268–76.

30. Lange KH, Andersen JL, Beyer N, et al. GH administration changes myosin heavy chain isoforms in skeletal muscle but does not augment muscle strength or hypertrophy, either alone or combined with resistance exercise training in healthy elderly men. J Clin Endocrinol Metab 2002;87(2):513–23.

31. Hennessey JV, Chromiak JA, DellaVentura S, et al. Growth hormone administration and exercise effects on muscle fiber type and diameter in moderately frail older people. J Am Geriatr Soc 2001;49(7):852–8.

32. Thompson JL, Butterfield GE, Gylfadottir UK, et al. Effects of human growth hormone, insulin-like growth factor I, and diet and exercise on body composition of obese postmenopausal women. J Clin Endocrinol Metab 1998;83(5):1477–84.

33. Hammarqvist F, Wennstrom I, Wernerman J. Effects of growth hormone and insulin-like growth factor-1 on postoperative muscle and substrate metabolism. J Nutr Metab 2010;2010. pii: 647929.

34. Welle S, Thornton C, Statt M, et al. Growth hormone increases muscle mass and strength but does not rejuvenate myofibrillar protein synthesis in healthy subjects over 60 years old. J Clin Endocrinol Metab 1996;81(9):3239–43.

35. Sugimoto T, Nakaoka D, Nasu M, et al. Effect of recombinant human growth hormone in elderly osteoporotic women. Clin Endocrinol (Oxf) 1999;51(6): 715–24.
36. Sattler FR, Castaneda-Sceppa C, Binder EF, et al. Testosterone and growth hormone improve body composition and muscle performance in older men. J Clin Endocrinol Metab 2009;94(6):1991–2001.
37. Blackman MR, Sorkin JD, Munzer T, et al. Growth hormone and sex steroid administration in healthy aged women and men: a randomized controlled trial. JAMA 2002;288(18):2282–92.
38. Brill KT, Weltman AL, Gentili A, et al. Single and combined effects of growth hormone and testosterone administration on measures of body composition, physical performance, mood, sexual function, bone turnover, and muscle gene expression in healthy older men. J Clin Endocrinol Metab 2002;87(12): 5649–57.
39. Nagaya N, Uematsu M, Kojima M, et al. Chronic administration of ghrelin improves left ventricular dysfunction and attenuates development of cardiac cachexia in rats with heart failure. Circulation 2001;104(12):1430–5.
40. Molfino A, Laviano A, Rossi Fanelli F. Contribution of anorexia to tissue wasting in cachexia. Curr Opin Support Palliat Care 2010;4(4):249–53.
41. Kung T, Springer J, Doehner W, et al. Novel treatment approaches to cachexia and sarcopenia: highlights from the 5th Cachexia Conference. Expert Opin Investig Drugs 2010;19(4):579–85.
42. Tai K, Visvanathan R, Hammond AJ, et al. Fasting ghrelin is related to skeletal muscle mass in healthy adults. Eur J Nutr 2009;48(3):176–83.
43. Nass R, Pezzoli SS, Oliveri MC, et al. Effects of an oral ghrelin mimetic on body composition and clinical outcomes in healthy older adults: a randomized trial. Ann Intern Med 2008;149(9):601–11.
44. Garcia JM, Polvino WJ. Effect on body weight and safety of RC-1291, a novel, orally available ghrelin mimetic and growth hormone secretagogue: results of a phase I, randomized, placebo-controlled, multiple-dose study in healthy volunteers. Oncologist 2007;12(5):594–600.
45. White HK, Petrie CD, Landschulz W, et al. Effects of an oral growth hormone secretagogue in older adults. J Clin Endocrinol Metab 2009;94(4):1198–206.
46. Farooqi IS, Keogh JM, Yeo GS, et al. Clinical spectrum of obesity and mutations in the melanocortin 4 receptor gene. N Engl J Med 2003;348(12):1085–95.
47. Scarlett JM, Bowe DD, Zhu X, et al. Genetic and pharmacologic blockade of central melanocortin signaling attenuates cardiac cachexia in rodent models of heart failure. J Endocrinol 2010;206(1):121–30.
48. von Haehling S, Stepney R, Anker SD. Advances in understanding and treating cardiac cachexia: highlights from the 5th Cachexia Conference. Int J Cardiol 2010;144(3):347–9.
49. Gallagher D, Visser M, De Meersman RE, et al. Appendicular skeletal muscle mass: effects of age, gender, and ethnicity. J Appl Physiol 1997;83(1):229–39.
50. Maltais ML, Desroches J, Dionne IJ. Changes in muscle mass and strength after menopause. J Musculoskelet Neuronal Interact 2009;9(4):186–97.
51. Jacobsen DE, Samson MM, Kezic S, et al. Postmenopausal HRT and tibolone in relation to muscle strength and body composition. Maturitas 2007;58(1):7–18.
52. Chlebowski RT, Schwartz AG, Wakelee H, et al. Oestrogen plus progestin and lung cancer in postmenopausal women (Women's Health Initiative trial): a post-hoc analysis of a randomised controlled trial. Lancet 2009;374(9697): 1243–51.

53. Meeuwsen IB, Samson MM, Duursma SA, et al. Muscle strength and tibolone: a randomised, double-blind, placebo-controlled trial. BJOG 2002;109(1): 77–84.

54. Meeuwsen IB, Samson MM, Duursma SA, et al. The effect of tibolone on fat mass, fat-free mass, and total body water in postmenopausal women. Endocrinology 2001;142(11):4813–7.

55. Arabi A, Garnero P, Porcher R, et al. Changes in body composition during post-menopausal hormone therapy: a 2 year prospective study. Hum Reprod 2003; 18(8):1747–52.

56. Hanggi W, Lippuner K, Jaeger P, et al. Differential impact of conventional oral or transdermal hormone replacement therapy or tibolone on body composition in postmenopausal women. Clin Endocrinol (Oxf) 1998;48(6):691–9.

57. Tommaselli GA, Di Carlo C, Di Spiezio Sardo A, et al. Serum leptin levels and body composition in postmenopausal women treated with tibolone and raloxifene. Menopause 2006;13(4):660–8.

58. Boyanov MA, Shinkov AD. Effects of tibolone on body composition in postmenopausal women: a 1-year follow up study. Maturitas 2005;51(4):363–9.

59. Welton AJ, Vickers MR, Kim J, et al. Health related quality of life after combined hormone replacement therapy: randomised controlled trial. BMJ 2008;337: a1190.

60. Lemoine S, Granier P, Tiffoche C, et al. Estrogen receptor alpha mRNA in human skeletal muscles. Med Sci Sports Exerc 2003;35(3):439–43.

61. Wiik A, Ekman M, Morgan G, et al. Oestrogen receptor beta is present in both muscle fibres and endothelial cells within human skeletal muscle tissue. Histochem Cell Biol 2005;124(2):161–5.

62. Dieli-Conwright CM, Spektor TM, Rice JC, et al. Influence of hormone replacement therapy on eccentric exercise induced myogenic gene expression in postmenopausal women. J Appl Physiol 2009;107(5):1381–8.

63. Dieli-Conwright CM, Spektor TM, Rice JC, et al. Hormone therapy attenuates exercise-induced skeletal muscle damage in postmenopausal women. J Appl Physiol 2009;107(3):853–8.

64. Huffman KM, Slentz CA, Johnson JL, et al. Impact of hormone replacement therapy on exercise training-induced improvements in insulin action in sedentary overweight adults. Metabolism 2008;57(7):888–95.

65. Sahu A. Minireview: a hypothalamic role in energy balance with special emphasis on leptin. Endocrinology 2004;145(6):2613–20.

66. Ceddia RB, William WN Jr, Curi R. The response of skeletal muscle to leptin. Front Biosci 2001;6:D90–7.

67. Trostler N, Romsos DR, Bergen WG, et al. Skeletal muscle accretion and turnover in lean and obese (ob/ob) mice. Metabolism 1979;28(9):928–33.

68. Sainz N, Rodriguez A, Catalan V, et al. Leptin administration favors muscle mass accretion by decreasing FoxO3a and increasing PGC-1alpha in ob/ob mice. PLoS One 2009;4(9):e6808.

69. Banks WA, Coon AB, Robinson SM, et al. Triglycerides induce leptin resistance at the blood-brain barrier. Diabetes 2004;53(5):1253–60.

70. Holick MF. The vitamin D deficiency pandemic and consequences for nonskeletal health: mechanisms of action. Mol Aspects Med 2008;29(6):361–8.

71. Morley JE. Vitamin d redux. J Am Med Dir Assoc 2009;10(9):591–2.

72. Braddy KK, Imam SN, Palla KR, et al. Vitamin d deficiency/insufficiency practice patterns in a veterans health administration long-term care population: a retrospective analysis. J Am Med Dir Assoc 2009;10(9):653–7.

73. Visser M, Deeg DJ, Lips P. Low vitamin D and high parathyroid hormone levels as determinants of loss of muscle strength and muscle mass (sarcopenia): the Longitudinal Aging Study Amsterdam. J Clin Endocrinol Metab 2003;88(12):5766–72.
74. Bischoff HA, Stahelin HB, Dick W, et al. Effects of vitamin D and calcium supplementation on falls: a randomized controlled trial. J Bone Miner Res 2003;18(2):343–51.
75. Pfeifer M, Begerow B, Minne HW, et al. Effects of a long-term vitamin D and calcium supplementation on falls and parameters of muscle function in community-dwelling older individuals. Osteoporos Int 2009;20(2):315–22.
76. Moreira-Pfrimer LD, Pedrosa MA, Teixeira L, et al. Treatment of vitamin D deficiency increases lower limb muscle strength in institutionalized older people independently of regular physical activity: a randomized double-blind controlled trial. Ann Nutr Metab 2009;54(4):291–300.
77. Pfeifer M, Begerow B, Minne HW, et al. Effects of a short-term vitamin D and calcium supplementation on body sway and secondary hyperparathyroidism in elderly women. J Bone Miner Res 2000;15(6):1113–8.
78. Bischoff-Ferrari HA, Orav EJ, Dawson-Hughes B. Effect of cholecalciferol plus calcium on falling in ambulatory older men and women: a 3-year randomized controlled trial. Arch Intern Med 2006;166(4):424–30.
79. Bischoff-Ferrari HA, Dawson-Hughes B, Staehelin HB, et al. Fall prevention with supplemental and active forms of vitamin D: a meta-analysis of randomised controlled trials. BMJ 2009;339:b3692.
80. Boland R. Role of vitamin D in skeletal muscle function. Endocr Rev 1986;7(4):434–48.
81. Wassner SJ, Li JB, Sperduto A, et al. Vitamin D Deficiency, hypocalcemia, and increased skeletal muscle degradation in rats. J Clin Invest 1983;72(1):102–12.
82. Janssen HC, Samson MM, Verhaar HJ. Vitamin D deficiency, muscle function, and falls in elderly people. Am J Clin Nutr 2002;75(4):611–5.
83. Sorensen OH, Lund B, Saltin B, et al. Myopathy in bone loss of ageing: improvement by treatment with 1 alpha-hydroxycholecalciferol and calcium. Clin Sci (Lond) 1979;56(2):157–61.
84. Ceglia L. Vitamin D and its role in skeletal muscle. Curr Opin Clin Nutr Metab Care 2009;12(6):628–33.
85. Bischoff HA, Borchers M, Gudat F, et al. In situ detection of 1,25-dihydroxyvitamin D3 receptor in human skeletal muscle tissue. Histochem J 2001;33(1):19–24.
86. Roth SM, Zmuda JM, Cauley JA, et al. Vitamin D receptor genotype is associated with fat-free mass and sarcopenia in elderly men. J Gerontol A Biol Sci Med Sci 2004;59(1):10–5.
87. Hamilton B. Vitamin D and human skeletal muscle. Scand J Med Sci Sports 2010;20(2):182–90.
88. Nguyen TM, Lieberherr M, Fritsch J, et al. The rapid effects of 1,25-dihydroxyvitamin D3 require the vitamin D receptor and influence 24-hydroxylase activity: studies in human skin fibroblasts bearing vitamin D receptor mutations. J Biol Chem 2004;279(9):7591–7.
89. Artaza JN, Bhasin S, Magee TR, et al. Myostatin inhibits myogenesis and promotes adipogenesis in C3H 10T(1/2) mesenchymal multipotent cells. Endocrinology 2005;146(8):3547–57.
90. Amirouche A, Durieux AC, Banzet S, et al. Down-regulation of Akt/mammalian target of rapamycin signaling pathway in response to myostatin overexpression in skeletal muscle. Endocrinology 2009;150(1):286–94.

91. Schuelke M, Wagner KR, Stolz LE, et al. Myostatin mutation associated with gross muscle hypertrophy in a child. N Engl J Med 2004;350(26):2682–8.
92. Siriett V, Salerno MS, Berry C, et al. Antagonism of myostatin enhances muscle regeneration during sarcopenia. Mol Ther 2007;15(8):1463–70.
93. Haidet AM, Rizo L, Handy C, et al. Long-term enhancement of skeletal muscle mass and strength by single gene administration of myostatin inhibitors. Proc Natl Acad Sci U S A 2008;105(11):4318–22.
94. Rodino-Klapac LR, Haidet AM, Kota J, et al. Inhibition of myostatin with emphasis on follistatin as a therapy for muscle disease. Muscle Nerve 2009; 39(3):283–96.
95. Tsuchida K. Targeting myostatin for therapies against muscle-wasting disorders. Curr Opin Drug Discov Devel 2008;11(4):487–94.
96. Solomon AM, Bouloux PM. Modifying muscle mass - the endocrine perspective. J Endocrinol 2006;191(2):349–60.
97. Nakatani M, Takehara Y, Sugino H, et al. Transgenic expression of a myostatin inhibitor derived from follistatin increases skeletal muscle mass and ameliorates dystrophic pathology in mdx mice. FASEB J 2008;22(2):477–87.
98. Ohsawa Y, Hagiwara H, Nakatani M, et al. Muscular atrophy of caveolin-3-deficient mice is rescued by myostatin inhibition. J Clin Invest 2006;116(11):2924–34.
99. Minetti GC, Colussi C, Adami R, et al. Functional and morphological recovery of dystrophic muscles in mice treated with deacetylase inhibitors. Nat Med 2006;12(10):1147–50.
100. Gilson H, Schakman O, Kalista S, et al. Follistatin induces muscle hypertrophy through satellite cell proliferation and inhibition of both myostatin and activin. Am J Physiol Endocrinol Metab 2009;297(1):E157–64.
101. Mendias CL, Bakhurin KI, Faulkner JA. Tendons of myostatin-deficient mice are small, brittle, and hypocellular. Proc Natl Acad Sci U S A 2008;105(1):388–93.
102. Savo A, Maiorano PM, Onder G, et al. Pharmacoepidemiology and disability in older adults: can medications slow the age-related decline in physical function? Expert Opin Pharmacother 2004;5(2):407–13.
103. Jones A, Woods DR. Skeletal muscle RAS and exercise performance. Int J Biochem Cell Biol 2003;35(6):855–66.
104. Onder G, Vedova CD, Pahor M. Effects of ACE inhibitors on skeletal muscle. Curr Pharm Des 2006;12(16):2057–64.
105. Sumukadas D, Witham MD, Struthers AD, et al. Ace inhibitors as a therapy for sarcopenia - evidence and possible mechanisms. J Nutr Health Aging 2008;12(7):480–5.
106. Onder G, Penninx BW, Balkrishnan R, et al. Relation between use of angiotensin-converting enzyme inhibitors and muscle strength and physical function in older women: an observational study. Lancet 2002;359(9310):926–30.
107. Di Bari M, van de Poll-Franse LV, Onder G, et al. Antihypertensive medications and differences in muscle mass in older persons: the health, aging and body composition study. J Am Geriatr Soc 2004;52(6):961–6.
108. Cesari M, Pedone C, Incalzi RA, et al. ACE-inhibition and physical function: results from the Trial of Angiotensin-Converting Enzyme Inhibition and Novel Cardiovascular Risk Factors (TRAIN) study. J Am Med Dir Assoc 2010;11(1):26–32.
109. Bunout D, Barrera G, de la Maza MP, et al. Effects of enalapril or nifedipine on muscle strength or functional capacity in elderly subjects. A double blind trial. J Renin Angiotensin Aldosterone Syst 2009;10(2):77–84.

110. Sumukadas D, Witham MD, Struthers AD, et al. Effect of perindopril on physical function in elderly people with functional impairment: a randomized controlled trial. CMAJ 2007;177(8):867–74.
111. Danser AH, Schalekamp MA, Bax WA, et al. Angiotensin-converting enzyme in the human heart. Effect of the deletion/insertion polymorphism. Circulation 1995; 92(6):1387–8.
112. Frederiksen H, Gaist D, Bathum L, et al. Angiotensin I-converting enzyme (ACE) gene polymorphism in relation to physical performance, cognition and survival–a follow-up study of elderly Danish twins. Ann Epidemiol 2003;13(1): 57–65.
113. Kritchevsky SB, Nicklas BJ, Visser M, et al. Angiotensin-converting enzyme insertion/deletion genotype, exercise, and physical decline. JAMA 2005;294(6):691–8.
114. Zhang B, Tanaka H, Shono N, et al. The I allele of the angiotensin-converting enzyme gene is associated with an increased percentage of slow-twitch type I fibers in human skeletal muscle. Clin Genet 2003;63(2):139–44.
115. Montgomery HE, Marshall R, Hemingway H, et al. Human gene for physical performance. Nature 1998;393(6682):221–2.
116. Williams AG, Rayson MP, Jubb M, et al. The ACE gene and muscle performance. Nature 2000;403(6770):614.
117. Montgomery H, Clarkson P, Barnard M, et al. Angiotensin-converting-enzyme gene insertion/deletion polymorphism and response to physical training. Lancet 1999;353(9152):541–5.
118. Vigano A, Trutschnigg B, Kilgour RD, et al. Relationship between angiotensin-converting enzyme gene polymorphism and body composition, functional performance, and blood biomarkers in advanced cancer patients. Clin Cancer Res 2009;15(7):2442–7.
119. Habouzit E, Richard H, Sanchez H, et al. Decreased muscle ACE activity enhances functional response to endurance training in rats, without change in muscle oxidative capacity or contractile phenotype. J Appl Physiol 2009;107(1):346–53.
120. Rizzoni D, Pasini E, Flati V, et al. Angiotensin receptor blockers improve insulin signaling and prevent microvascular rarefaction in the skeletal muscle of spontaneously hypertensive rats. J Hypertens 2008;26(8):1595–601.
121. Guo Q, Minami N, Mori N, et al. Effects of estradiol, angiotensin-converting enzyme inhibitor and exercise training on exercise capacity and skeletal muscle in old female rats. Clin Exp Hypertens 2010;32(2):76–83.
122. Takeshita S, Tomiyama H, Yokoyama N, et al. Angiotensin-converting enzyme inhibition improves defective angiogenesis in the ischemic limb of spontaneously hypertensive rats. Cardiovasc Res 2001;52(2):314–20.
123. Weisinger RS, Stanley TK, Begg DP, et al. Angiotensin converting enzyme inhibition lowers body weight and improves glucose tolerance in C57BL/6J mice maintained on a high fat diet. Physiol Behav 2009;98(1–2):192–7.
124. Clerk LH, Vincent MA, Barrett EJ, et al. Skeletal muscle capillary responses to insulin are abnormal in late-stage diabetes and are restored by angiotensin-converting enzyme inhibition. Am J Physiol Endocrinol Metab 2007;293(6): E1804–9.
125. Han Y, Runge MS, Brasier AR. Angiotensin II induces interleukin-6 transcription in vascular smooth muscle cells through pleiotropic activation of nuclear factor-kappa B transcription factors. Circ Res 1999;84(6):695–703.
126. Kranzhofer R, Schmidt J, Pfeiffer CA, et al. Angiotensin induces inflammatory activation of human vascular smooth muscle cells. Arterioscler Thromb Vasc Biol 1999;19(7):1623–9.

127. Browatzki M, Larsen D, Pfeiffer CA, et al. Angiotensin II stimulates matrix metal-loproteinase secretion in human vascular smooth muscle cells via nuclear factor-kappaB and activator protein 1 in a redox-sensitive manner. J Vasc Res 2005;42(5):415–23.

128. Payne GW. Effect of inflammation on the aging microcirculation: impact on skeletal muscle blood flow control. Microcirculation 2006;13(4):343–52.

129. Brull DJ, Sanders J, Rumley A, et al. Impact of angiotensin converting enzyme inhibition on post-coronary artery bypass interleukin 6 release. Heart 2002; 87(3):252–5.

130. Tian Q, Miyazaki R, Ichiki T, et al. Inhibition of tumor necrosis factor-alpha-induced interleukin-6 expression by telmisartan through cross-talk of peroxisome proliferator-activated receptor-gamma with nuclear factor kappaB and CCAAT/enhancer-binding protein-beta. Hypertension 2009;53(5):798–804.

131. Fujita K, Yoneda M, Wada K, et al. Telmisartan, an angiotensin II type 1 receptor blocker, controls progress of nonalcoholic steatohepatitis in rats. Dig Dis Sci 2007;52(12):3455–64.

132. Sugimoto K, Kazdova L, Qi NR, et al. Telmisartan increases fatty acid oxidation in skeletal muscle through a peroxisome proliferator-activated receptor-gamma dependent pathway. J Hypertens 2008;26(6):1209–15.

133. Giovannini S, Marzetti E, Borst SE, et al. Modulation of GH/IGF-1 axis: potential strategies to counteract sarcopenia in older adults. Mech Ageing Dev 2008; 129(10):593–601.

134. Musaro A, McCullagh KJ, Naya FJ, et al. IGF-1 induces skeletal myocyte hyper-trophy through calcineurin in association with GATA-2 and NF-ATc1. Nature 1999;400(6744):581–5.

135. Brink M, Price SR, Chrast J, et al. Angiotensin II induces skeletal muscle wasting through enhanced protein degradation and down-regulates autocrine insulin-like growth factor I. Endocrinology 2001;142(4):1489–96.

136. Onder G, Liperoti R, Russo A, et al. Use of ACE inhibitors is associated with elevated levels of IGFBP-3 among hypertensive older adults: results from the II-SIRENTE study. Eur J Clin Pharmacol 2007;63(4):389–95.

137. Maggio M, Ceda GP, Lauretani F, et al. Relation of angiotensin-converting enzyme inhibitor treatment to insulin-like growth factor-1 serum levels in subjects >65 years of age (the InCHIANTI study). Am J Cardiol 2006;97(10):1525–9.

138. Armitage J, Bowman L, Collins R, et al. Effects of simvastatin 40 mg daily on muscle and liver adverse effects in a 5-year randomized placebo-controlled trial in 20,536 high-risk people. BMC Clin Pharmacol 2009;9:6.

139. Robinson MM, Hamilton KL, Miller BF. The interactions of some commonly consumed drugs with mitochondrial adaptations to exercise. J Appl Physiol 2009;107(1):8–16.

140. Scott D, Blizzard L, Fell J, et al. Statin therapy, muscle function and falls risk in community-dwelling older adults. QJM 2009;102(9):625–33.

141. Giri J, McDermott MM, Greenland P, et al. Statin use and functional decline in patients with and without peripheral arterial disease. J Am Coll Cardiol 2006; 47(5):998–1004.

142. Agostini JV, Tinetti ME, Han L, et al. Effects of statin use on muscle strength, cognition, and depressive symptoms in older adults. J Am Geriatr Soc 2007; 55(3):420–5.

143. LaCroix AZ, Gray SL, Aragaki A, et al. Statin use and incident frailty in women aged 65 years or older: prospective findings from the Women's Health Initiative Observational Study. J Gerontol A Biol Sci Med Sci 2008;63(4):369–75.

144. Riechman SE, Andrews RD, Maclean DA, et al. Statins and dietary and serum cholesterol are associated with increased lean mass following resistance training. J Gerontol A Biol Sci Med Sci 2007;62(10):1164–71.
145. Clough GF, Turzyniecka M, Walter L, et al. Muscle microvascular dysfunction in central obesity is related to muscle insulin insensitivity but is not reversed by high-dose statin treatment. Diabetes 2009;58(5):1185–91.
146. Thompson PD, Parker BA, Clarkson PM, et al. A randomized clinical trial to assess the effect of statins on skeletal muscle function and performance: rationale and study design. Prev Cardiol 2010;13(3):104–11.
147. Ades PA, Gunther PG, Meyer WL, et al. Cardiac and skeletal muscle adaptations to training in systemic hypertension and effect of beta blockade (metoprolol or propranolol). Am J Cardiol 1990;66(5):591–6.
148. Langin D. Adipose tissue lipolysis as a metabolic pathway to define pharmacological strategies against obesity and the metabolic syndrome. Pharmacol Res 2006;53(6):482–91.
149. Dalla Libera L, Ravara B, Gobbo V, et al. Skeletal muscle proteins oxidation in chronic right heart failure in rats: can different beta-blockers prevent it to the same degree? Int J Cardiol 2010;143(2):192–9.
150. Scherrer U, Randin D, Vollenweider P, et al. Nitric oxide release accounts for insulin's vascular effects in humans. J Clin Invest 1994;94(6):2511–5.
151. Steinberg HO, Brechtel G, Johnson A, et al. Insulin-mediated skeletal muscle vasodilation is nitric oxide dependent. A novel action of insulin to increase nitric oxide release. J Clin Invest 1994;94(3):1172–9.
152. Timmerman KL, Lee JL, Fujita S, et al. Pharmacological vasodilation improves insulin-stimulated muscle protein anabolism but not glucose utilization in older adults. Diabetes 2010;59(11):2764–71.
153. Meneilly GS, Elliot T, Bryer-Ash M, et al. Insulin-mediated increase in blood flow is impaired in the elderly. J Clin Endocrinol Metab 1995;80(6):1899–903.
154. Rasmussen BB, Fujita S, Wolfe RR, et al. Insulin resistance of muscle protein metabolism in aging. FASEB J 2006;20(6):768–9.
155. Sindler AL, Delp MD, Reyes R, et al. Effects of ageing and exercise training on eNOS uncoupling in skeletal muscle resistance arterioles. J Physiol 2009; 587(Pt 15):3885–97.
156. Haslett P, Hempstead M, Seidman C, et al. The metabolic and immunologic effects of short-term thalidomide treatment of patients infected with the human immunodeficiency virus. AIDS Res Hum Retroviruses 1997;13(12): 1047–54.
157. Steffen BT, Lees SJ, Booth FW. Anti-TNF treatment reduces rat skeletal muscle wasting in monocrotaline-induced cardiac cachexia. J Appl Physiol 2008; 105(6):1950–8.
158. Calabrese LH, Zein N, Vassilopoulos D. Safety of antitumour necrosis factor (anti-TNF) therapy in patients with chronic viral infections: hepatitis C, hepatitis B, and HIV infection. Ann Rheum Dis 2004;63(Suppl 2):ii18–24.
159. Ruxton CH, Reed SC, Simpson MJ, et al. The health benefits of omega-3 polyunsaturated fatty acids: a review of the evidence. J Hum Nutr Diet 2004;17(5): 449–59.
160. Stillwell W, Wassall SR. Docosahexaenoic acid: membrane properties of a unique fatty acid. Chem Phys Lipids 2003;126(1):1–27.
161. Haugaard SB, Vaag A, Mu H, et al. Skeletal muscle structural lipids improve during weight-maintenance after a very low calorie dietary intervention. Lipids Health Dis 2009;8:34.

162. Maillet D, Weber JM. Relationship between n-3 PUFA content and energy metabolism in the flight muscles of a migrating shorebird: evidence for natural doping. J Exp Biol 2007;210(Pt 3):413–20.

163. Barber MD, Ross JA, Voss AC, et al. The effect of an oral nutritional supplement enriched with fish oil on weight-loss in patients with pancreatic cancer. Br J Cancer 1999;81(1):80–6.

164. Broekhuizen R, Wouters EF, Creutzberg EC, et al. Polyunsaturated fatty acids improve exercise capacity in chronic obstructive pulmonary disease. Thorax 2005;60(5):376–82.

165. Robinson SM, Jameson KA, Batelaan SF, et al. Diet and its relationship with grip strength in community-dwelling older men and women: the Hertfordshire cohort study. J Am Geriatr Soc 2008;56(1):84–90.

166. Rousseau JH, Kleppinger A, Kenny AM. Self-reported dietary intake of omega-3 fatty acids and association with bone and lower extremity function. J Am Geriatr Soc 2009;57(10):1781–8.

167. Calder PC. n-3 polyunsaturated fatty acids, inflammation, and inflammatory diseases. Am J Clin Nutr 2006;83(Suppl 6):1505S–19S.

168. Smith GI, Atherton P, Reeds DN, et al. Dietary omega-3 fatty acid supplementation increases the rate of muscle protein synthesis in older adults: a randomized controlled trial. Am J Clin Nutr 2011;93(2):402–12.

169. Coll T, Alvarez-Guardia D, Barroso E, et al. Activation of peroxisome proliferator-activated receptor-{delta} by GW501516 prevents fatty acid-induced nuclear factor-{kappa}B activation and insulin resistance in skeletal muscle cells. Endocrinology 2010;151(4):1560–9.

170. Trappe TA, Carroll CC, Dickinson JM, et al. Influence of acetaminophen and ibuprofen on skeletal muscle adaptations to resistance exercise in older adults. Am J Physiol Regul Integr Comp Physiol 2011;300(3):R655–62.

171. Brose A, Parise G, Tarnopolsky MA. Creatine supplementation enhances isometric strength and body composition improvements following strength exercise training in older adults. J Gerontol A Biol Sci Med Sci 2003;58(1):11–9.

172. Jones AM, Wilkerson DP, Fulford J. Influence of dietary creatine supplementation on muscle phosphocreatine kinetics during knee-extensor exercise in humans. Am J Physiol Regul Integr Comp Physiol 2009;296(4):R1078–87.

173. Chrusch MJ, Chilibeck PD, Chad KE, et al. Creatine supplementation combined with resistance training in older men. Med Sci Sports Exerc 2001;33(12):2111–7.

174. Rawson ES, Wehnert ML, Clarkson PM. Effects of 30 days of creatine ingestion in older men. Eur J Appl Physiol Occup Physiol 1999;80(2):139–44.

175. Bermon S, Venembre P, Sachet C, et al. Effects of creatine monohydrate ingestion in sedentary and weight-trained older adults. Acta Physiol Scand 1998; 164(2):147–55.

176. Jakobi JM, Rice CL, Curtin SV, et al. Neuromuscular properties and fatigue in older men following acute creatine supplementation. Eur J Appl Physiol 2001; 84(4):321–8.

177. Rawson ES, Clarkson PM. Acute creatine supplementation in older men. Int J Sports Med 2000;21(1):71–5.

178. Stout JR, Sue Graves B, Cramer JT, et al. Effects of creatine supplementation on the onset of neuromuscular fatigue threshold and muscle strength in elderly men and women (64–86 years). J Nutr Health Aging 2007;11(6):459–64.

179. Tarnopolsky M, Zimmer A, Paikin J, et al. Creatine monohydrate and conjugated linoleic acid improve strength and body composition following resistance exercise in older adults. PLoS One 2007;2(10):e991.

180. Burke DG, Chilibeck PD, Parise G, et al. Effect of creatine and weight training on muscle creatine and performance in vegetarians. Med Sci Sports Exerc 2003; 35(11):1946–55.

181. Candow DG, Little JP, Chilibeck PD, et al. Low-dose creatine combined with protein during resistance training in older men. Med Sci Sports Exerc 2008; 40(9):1645–52.

182. Willoughby DS, Rosene JM. Effects of oral creatine and resistance training on myogenic regulatory factor expression. Med Sci Sports Exerc 2003;35(6):923–9.

183. Parise G, Mihic S, MacLennan D, et al. Effects of acute creatine monohydrate supplementation on leucine kinetics and mixed-muscle protein synthesis. J Appl Physiol 2001;91(3):1041–7.

184. Sestili P, Martinelli C, Bravi G, et al. Creatine supplementation affords cytoprotection in oxidatively injured cultured mammalian cells via direct antioxidant activity. Free Radic Biol Med 2006;40(5):837–49.

185. Balsom PD, Soderlund K, Sjodin B, et al. Skeletal muscle metabolism during short duration high-intensity exercise: influence of creatine supplementation. Acta Physiol Scand 1995;154(3):303–10.

186. Francaux M, Poortmans JR. Effects of training and creatine supplement on muscle strength and body mass. Eur J Appl Physiol Occup Physiol 1999; 80(2):165–8.

187. Olsen S, Aagaard P, Kadi F, et al. Creatine supplementation augments the increase in satellite cell and myonuclei number in human skeletal muscle induced by strength training. J Physiol 2006;573(Pt 2):525–34.

188. Dawson-Hughes B, Castaneda-Sceppa C, Harris SS, et al. Impact of supplementation with bicarbonate on lower-extremity muscle performance in older men and women. Osteoporos Int 2010;21(7):1171–9.

189. Cao Z, Wu Y, Curry K, et al. Ginkgo biloba extract EGb 761 and Wisconsin Ginseng delay sarcopenia in Caenorhabditis elegans. J Gerontol A Biol Sci Med Sci 2007;62(12):1337–45.

190. Bidon C, Lachuer J, Molgo J, et al. The extract of Ginkgo biloba EGb 761 reactivates a juvenile profile in the skeletal muscle of sarcopenic rats by transcriptional reprogramming. PLoS One 2009;4(11):e7998.

191. Xu J, Seo AY, Vorobyeva DA, et al. Beneficial effects of a Q-ter based nutritional mixture on functional performance, mitochondrial function, and oxidative stress in rats. PLoS One 2010;5(5):e10572.

192. Sumien N, Heinrich KR, Shetty RA, et al. Prolonged intake of coenzyme Q10 impairs cognitive functions in mice. J Nutr 2009;139(10):1926–32.

193. Abellan van Kan G, Rolland YM, Morley JE, et al. Frailty: toward a clinical definition. J Am Med Dir Assoc 2008;9(2):71–2.

194. Morley JE, Kim MJ, Haren MT, et al. Frailty and the aging male. Aging Male 2005;8(3–4):135–40.

Physical Activity and Sarcopenia

Fabien Pillard, MD, PhD[a,b,c,*], Dalila Laoudj-Chenivesse, PhD[d,e],
Gilles Carnac, PhD[d], Jacques Mercier, MD, PhD[d,e,f],
Jacques Rami, PhD[a,b,c], Daniel Rivière, MD, PhD[a,b,c],
Yves Rolland, MD, PhD[g,h,i]

KEYWORDS

• Exercise prescription • Exercise intensity • Training

Multiple factors and mechanisms contribute to the age-related impairment of the function and mass of the skeletal skinned muscles that indicates the diagnosis of sarcopenia. Recent longitudinal aging studies suggest that sarcopenia may be secondary to muscle weakness in the elderly (see Refs.[1,2] for reviews). These recent studies, as well as the work of a research group on sarcopenia 10 years previously,[3] also demonstrated that muscle strength, but not muscle mass, is independently associated with lower extremity performance, another factor for disability among older persons. As exercise training enhances muscle mass and function in nonelderly subjects and as lack of activity (or inactivity) is an important contributor to loss of muscle mass and strength at any age,[4–7] it is of interest to examine whether physical activity, a functional therapy and a modifiable lifestyle behavior, could be proposed in treatment and prevention of sarcopenia, which is in part a functional disease. In the present article the authors first briefly show how physical activity may alter muscle properties in sarcopenia, then examine its evidence-based clinical effect on sarcopenia. The principles governing the prescription of physical activity for subjects with sarcopenia are also

The authors have no conflicts of interest to report.

[a] Respiratory Exploration Department and Sports Medicine Department, Larrey University Hospital, 24 chemin de Pouvourville, 31059, Toulouse CEDEX 9, France
[b] Physiology Department, Medical University of Toulouse III, France
[c] French National Institute for Health and Medical Research (INSERM), Obesity Research Unit U858 - I2MR, Toulouse, France
[d] French National Institute for Health and Medical Research (INSERM), ERI 25, Montpellier 34000, France
[e] Medical University of Montpellier, EA-4202, Montpellier, France
[f] University Hospital of Montpellier, France
[g] National Institute for Health and Medical Research (INSERM), U558, Toulouse, France
[h] Medical University of Toulouse III, France
[i] Department of Geriatric Medicine, University Hospital of Toulouse, France
* Corresponding author. Service d'Exploration de la Fonction Respiratoire et de Médecine du Sport, CHU Larrey, 24 chemin de Pouvourville, 31059, Toulouse CEDEX 9, France.
E-mail address: fpillard@hotmail.com

discussed. The factors that can be modified by physical training and the principles on which prescription should be based are summarized in **Fig. 1.**

PHYSICAL ACTIVITY FOR SARCOPENIA: FROM HUMAN TO CELL

Age-related changes in skeletal skinned muscle can largely be attributed to the interaction of factors affecting neuromuscular transmission, muscle (and tendon) architecture, fiber composition, excitation-contraction coupling, and metabolism. Before aging exerts its influence, muscle fibers display plasticity of their biochemical and morphologic properties when they are exposed to different functional demands. Throughout the human aging process, the loss of strength in old age is predominantly accounted for by reduced muscle mass and myofibrillar protein content in consequence of a combination of progressive fiber loss and fiber atrophy. The aging process is often characterized by investigators as a selective loss of fast-twitch fibers in muscle.[8] However, when electrophoretic and not histochemical identification of muscle fiber phenotype was performed, other studies indicated that the distribution of fiber types is relatively stable across the aging part of the life span, in particular because of the identification of a high percentage of hybrid fibers (coexpressing more than one myosin heavy chain isoform).[9] However, despite aging, sarcopenia, and significant functional alterations of the overall muscle, the contractile function of surviving fibers may be preserved in older humans as suggested by the upregulation of basal levels of some myogenic regulation factors (MRFs),[10–12] and by the link between upregulation and the degree of sarcopenia in rodents.[13] These findings suggest that surviving fibers are still prone to plasticity in response to different functional demands such as physical exercise; this response helps elderly muscle to compensate to partially correct muscle size deficit in an attempt to maintain optimal force-generating capacity.[14] Regular physical activity can thus partially correct the acceleration of sarcopenic progression related to inactivity and poor nutrition.[15]

From an overall viewpoint, the quantitative aspect of sarcopenia is attributable to an imbalance between protein synthesis and degradation or between apoptosis and regeneration processes, or both. The influence of physical activity in sarcopenic muscle can be described in relation to several of the factors acting on muscle in age-related imbalance processes.

Effect of Physical Activity on Muscle Anabolism in Elderly Subjects

A key intracellular pathway that coordinates signals in the regulation of muscle protein synthesis is the mammalian target of rapamycin (mTOR), which plays a key regulatory role in the regulation of translation initiation.[16] Following acute exercise in animals and young humans, components of the mTOR pathway are rapidly upregulated (see Ref.[17] for review, and Ref.[18]), but little is known of changes in mTOR activity and total protein content with chronic exercise. On the other hand, there are only indirect data suggesting positive mTOR signaling mechanisms in aged human skeletal muscle following exercise.[19,20] A reduction in myostatin gene expression (a negative regulatory factor of skeletal muscle development) in older as well as in young subjects could also influence anabolic response following exercise in older persons.[12] Serum myostatin-immunoreactive protein levels have been found to be higher in 60- to 75-year-old men and women than in younger 19- to 35-year-olds, and were inversely correlated with muscle mass corrected for height.[21] Whatever the pathway, Kosek and colleagues[22] suggested that the effective, but lower, anabolic muscle response in older than in young men after a 16-week resistance training program, 3 days a week, was not explained by age-related variation in the expression of myogenic

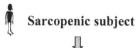 **Sarcopenic subject**

⇩

Sarcopenic skinned skeletal muscle cells

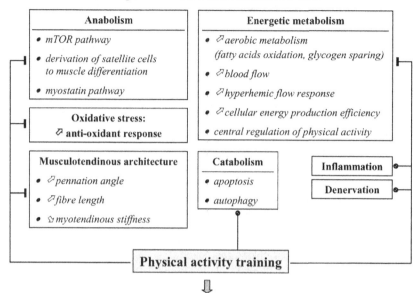

Anabolism	Energetic metabolism
• mTOR pathway	• ⬈aerobic metabolism (fatty acids oxidation, glycogen sparing)
• derivation of satellite cells to muscle differentiation	• ⬈blood flow
• myostatin pathway	• ⬈hyperhemic flow response
Oxidative stress: ⬈ anti-oxidant response	• ⬈cellular energy production efficiency
	• central regulation of physical activity

Musculotendinous architecture	Catabolism	Inflammation
• ⬈pennation angle	• apoptosis	Denervation
• ⬈fibre length	• autophagy	
• ⬉myotendinous stiffness		

Physical activity training

⇩

Prescription of physical activity; defining:

• the drug, i.e. the physical activity agent

• the dose of physical activity that must be delivered (intensity ✕ time)

• the frequency of the administration of physical activity

• the context of the administration of physical activity (who monitors PA sessions?)

Recommended prescription

• resistance training (and eccentric exercises)

• endurance training   **Physically active lifestyle and codified exercise**

• (low intensity occlusion training)

⇩

Evidence based epidemiological effect of physical activity training on sarcopenia: it's never too late!

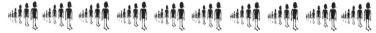

Fig. 1. Summary of the association between sarcopenia and physical activity training. ⊢ Positive modulation; —◉ negative modulation.

regulation factors. One explanation was that the RNA-to-protein ratio is higher in old than in young muscles, suggesting a decrease in translational efficiency over the life span. Finally, transcription-mediated effects of physical activity leading to satellite cell activation and proliferation factors could be useful to divert satellite cells to muscle differentiation and not adipocyte differentiation,[23] because failure to express the transcription factors that direct muscle mesenchymal precursors into fully differentiated functionally specialized cells may be responsible for their phenotypic switch into the adipogenic lineage (see Ref.[24] for review).

Although both young and elderly humans show an increase in some muscle factors associated with proliferation and differentiation, and a reduction in myostatin gene expression following exercise, the quantitative anabolic response to resistance exercise (protein mass) is lower in the elderly than in the young. Some investigators consider that this could be linked with the opposing and higher expression of proteolytic regulators (see Ref.[25] for review), whereas according to other investigators upregulation of atrophy gene expression does not seem to be involved in the sarcopenia process.[26] When interpreting discrepancies of results between investigators, one should bear in mind that both animal and human studies are performed with the common aim of identifying a strategic axis for the management of sarcopenia in humans. Increased apoptosis is another and negative process that has been identified as a possible pathway leading to the development of sarcopenia; as a countermeasure against apoptosis, it has been suggested that increased chronic activity attenuates apoptotic signaling and may reduce sarcopenia in rats.[27,28] In rodent skeletal muscle, exercise associated with mild caloric restriction may also attenuate the age-related impairment of autophagy (a process of degradation of cellular constituents, that when controlled could be a useful mechanism to combat cell damage and death).[29]

Upstream of the intracellular pathways coordinating muscle protein anabolism in older subjects, some hormones might influence this response of muscle to exercise. Wilkes and colleagues[30] recently suggested that blunting of insulin inhibition of proteolysis in legs of older subjects may contribute to age-related sarcopenia, and that this effect may be mediated through blunted Akt-PKB activation. As exercise training enhances insulin sensitivity in older subjects,[31] and according to the authors' previous hypothesis may have a positive effect on mTOR signaling mechanisms, it may also have a positive effect on the sarcopenic process by enhancing insulin inhibition of proteolysis. Androgenic response to exercise has also been hypothesized as a hormonal mechanism explaining muscle response to exercise. In a recent study, Ahtiainen and colleagues[32] demonstrated in older men that a 21-week long program of strength, endurance, or combined training specifically increased strength and muscle mass as well as aerobic capacity according to the training method, but no significant relationship was shown between these functional adaptations and androgenic response, that is, serum testosterone or cytoplasmic androgen receptor (AR) concentration measured 4 to 5 days after the last training session. This result is in contradiction with the association between androgenic and functional clinical responses observed after exercise and described in other studies[33-35] but, unlike Ahtiainen's study, these were not performed in elderly subjects and the biological response was evaluated very shortly after the stimulation by muscular exercise. Moreover, as suggested by these investigators, the testosterone effect may be affected by nongenomic signaling mechanisms through transmembrane G-protein–coupled receptors and linked to an increase in free Ca^{2+} and activation of mitogen-activated protein kinase,[36] which are signaling pathways in the development of skeletal muscle hypertrophy.[37] Lastly, the subjects evaluated in the study of Ahtiainen and colleagues had normal plasma testosterone concentrations before starting the physical activity program, so the potential variation of this biological parameter in relation to baseline level was smaller. Physical activity could thus have a favorable effect on the "muscle testosterone axis" in subjects with low plasma levels of this hormone, as does testosterone supplementation in the same subjects. Even according to this hypothesis, exercise-mediated androgenic pathway activation may not sufficiently explain the effect of exercise on functional parameters, as there are conflicting and inconclusive results on the effectiveness of testosterone therapy on muscle mass and muscle strength in the elderly, even in hypogonadal subjects. However, no study has used androgen supplementation combined with exercise training to examine how these two treatment methods could each potentialize the other (see Ref.[38] for review). Such a synergistic effect between exercise and hormone replacement therapy (HRT) has been suggested for estrogen replacement therapy in a randomized controlled trial in middle-aged women in early menopause: additional exercise resulted in additive or even synergistic effects of HRT on muscle (evaluated by vertical jumping height and relative proportion of fat within the muscle compartment).[39] A third "hormonal" response of muscle to exercise training relates to the insulin-like growth factor 1 (IGF-1) pathway. IGF-1 is a potent mitogen and anabolic agent that plays an important role in the growth of various body tissues, including skeletal muscle. The decline of circulating IGF-1 levels with advancing age is also related to loss of muscle mass and strength. Strength training has been reported to increase the skeletal muscle fraction of IGF-1 protein and muscle IGF-1 mRNA levels, that is, the noncirculating fraction of this factor, even in the elderly.[40,41] It has been suggested that IGF-1 gene polymorphisms influence muscle phenotypic responses to strength training in older men and women,[42] which could explain why the phenotypic and functional effects of such training on muscle differ between studies.

As a nonspecific cellular pathway and in addition to contractile activity, feeding increases the rate of protein synthesis compared with the unfed state. This process appears to be mainly caused by increased amino acid availability (particularly essential amino acids) rather than feeding-induced increase in insulin concentrations[43] (see the article Nutrition and Sarcopenia by Volpi and colleagues elsewhere in this issue of the journal).

Effect of Physical Activity on Muscle Energetic Metabolism in Elderly Subjects

Whether or not one considers that the sarcopenic process may be characterized by selective atrophy of type II muscle fibers, both type I and type II fibers are affected by metabolic dysfunction in the context of sarcopenia.

In healthy older adults, there is evidence of mitochondrial impairment and muscle weakness, but functional indicators of impairment, such as phosphodiester enhancement in muscle, can be reversed and the transcriptome enhanced, resulting in improvement of the sarcopenic muscle phenotype when subjects are physically active.[44–47] What remains less clear is whether the decline in skeletal muscle mitochondrial oxidative capacity is purely a function of the aging process, or whether the sedentary lifestyle of the elderly subjects studied acts as a confounder in the association between these two factors.

As oxygen availability for mitochondria is a potential limiting factor of aerobic metabolism, reduced muscle capillarity, decreased maximal blood flow, slower hyperemic flow response,[48,49] arterial stifness,[50] and disruption of the microvascular endothelium[51] have been reported in some studies in sedentary older people, but not in all. Exercise training can improve these functions and so could limit at cellular level the mitochondrial dysfunction in sarcopenic muscle. Finally, Chow and colleagues[52] highlighted that exercise training increased spontaneous physical activity (as measured with infrared photocell sensors) in a murine model. Despite the fact that this model was murine and that the rodents were not old, this change could have important implications for aging, because it supports the notion of a relation between mitochondrial function and spontaneous physical activity, and suggests that exercise training may be a viable approach to interruption of the vicious cycle of aging.

When muscular oxidative capacity drops, anaerobic metabolism is more able to sustain energy (adenosine triphosphate [ATP]) production, in particular when exercise intensity increases as in resistance exercise: glycogen then becomes an essential substrate for energy production while fatty acid use decreases. Looking beyond the defect in mitochondrial function, the decrease in resting muscle glycogen concentration after use is not favorable to resistance exercise in older humans. As previously stated, endurance training can reverse mitochondrial dysfunction and so contribute to reduce glycogen depletion because it enhances fatty acids oxidation, making glycogen available for resistance exercise.[53] Notwithstanding the restoration of oxidative metabolism and the consequent sparing of glycogen, energy supply is limited by the availability of substrates. Fatty acids, proteins, and carbohydrates can be oxidized by muscle, but fatty acids are preferential substrates until the energy output supplied matches with the energy output of muscular contraction, which occurs at low to moderate intensities of endurance exercise.[54] Sufficient fatty acid oxidation is also of interest because excess fatty acids can limit glycolysis through the Randle cycle[55] and so supply energy for high-intensity exercise (relative to the maximal intensity). It has been suggested that the availability of muscle carnitine (a substrate for carnitine palmitoyl-transferase that transports acetyl-coenzyme A into mitochondria) may limit fatty acid oxidation. As there seems to be a negative correlation between advancing age and muscle carnitine levels, carnitine deficiency may therefore contribute to geriatric frailty (see Ref.[56] for review). However, endurance training can reverse carnitine dysfunction in humans, as described by Lanza and colleagues,[31] who showed in young (18–30 years old) as well as in old subjects (59–76 years old) that endurance training was associated with better ATP production through the carnitine pathway and increased muscular oxidative capacity. In rats, upregulation of uncoupling protein 3 (UCP3) in aged muscle also limited ATP-generating capacity of the fiber.[57] Exercise training could be suggested as a countermeasure to restore cellular energy production efficiency, as training decreased UCP3 protein levels in young untrained subjects.[58] This last assumption needs to be tested for sarcopenia in elderly individuals. Training also elicits (restores) UCP3 content in limb muscle of patients with chronic obstructive pulmonary disease, and it has been hypothesized that UCP3 may protect muscle against lipotoxicity (also detrimental to muscle function in sarcopenia).[59]

Another consequence of the mitochondrial dysfunction could be the alteration of the central regulation of physical activity (see Ref.[8] for details). It is has been suggested that spontaneous physical activity is regulated by hypothalamic centers in response to signals from the peripheral tissues, especially from skeletal muscle mitochondrial ATP. If mitochondrial ATP production in peripheral skeletal muscle declines, thus downregulating activity levels via efferent sympathetic or chemical signals, spontaneous activity would lessen with age in response to declining mitochondrial function in peripheral tissue. Moreover, it has been suggested that reduced spontaneous activity and other unknown regulatory factors interact to reduce the cognitive phenomenon of "motivation" in older persons to engage in voluntary physical activity. According to this model, both spontaneous and voluntary physical activities decrease with age as a result of the alteration of mitochondrial ATP production. Exercise training could then stimulate spontaneous physical activity and motivation in the elderly through its positive effect on the mitochondrial function.

Effect of Physical Activity on Oxidative Stress in Elderly Subjects

The level of oxidative stress imposed on cells is influenced by two fundamental biological processes: increased generation of reactive oxygen species (ROS) and decreased generation of antioxidant defense. During aging, as in exposed young subjects, increased oxidative stress in skeletal muscle leads to the accumulation of damaged proteins, which are not properly eliminated, aggregate, and in turn impair proteolytic activities.[60] Myocytes, satellite cells (SCs),[61] neuromuscular junction, and mitochondria[62] are damaged by oxidative stress, and have been depicted as potential mechanisms of sarcopenia. Mitochondrial ROS production is a factor that could be implicated in the adipogenic conversion of SCs.[24] An association between skeletal muscle weakness and oxidative stress has been confirmed in a cohort study conducted over 36 months in a large (N = 545) sample of American women older than 65 years (the Women's Health and Aging Study I). After adjusting for confounding variables, serum protein carbonyls (markers of oxidative damages to proteins) were associated with a decline in walking speed over 36 months and with incident severe walking disability (hazard ratio 1.42, 95% confidence interval 1.02–1.98).[63]

Mitochondria are damaged by ROS but also produce them, leading to an adaptive response that subsequently increases stress resistance. This response is assumed to reduce oxidative stress in the long term when in contact with ROS. This type of retrograde response has been named mitochondrial hormesis or mitohormesis, and may in addition be applicable to the health-promoting effects of physical exercise in humans.[64] The challenge is then to stimulate mitohormesis against sarcopenia by exercise, as this alters mitochondrial function. Although gene expression of some antioxidant enzymes can be enhanced after an acute bout of exercise, the consecutive increase in de novo protein synthesis of an antioxidant enzyme usually requires repeated bouts of exercise. Moreover, according to the concept of "oxidative stress homeostasis," nonexhaustive exercise can induce mild stress that stimulates the expression of certain antioxidant enzymes, although this training-induced adaptation seems to be attenuated by aging.[65] Targeting oxidative stress with exercise through an antioxidant response seems rational in fighting against age-induced muscle performance impairment that occurs with or without sarcopenia. However, it has recently been suggested that training should be supplemented by exogenous antioxidants to seek the optimal level of defense.

Effect of Physical Activity on Muscle Inflammation in Elderly Subjects

Inflammation may be a potential factor in the development of sarcopenia through stimulation of proteolytic signaling. Recent evidence indicates that chronic resistance training contributes to the control of locally derived inflammation via adaptations to repeated and acute increases in proinflammatory mRNA within muscle.[66] Exercise-induced changes in heat-shock protein (Hsp), responsible for cellular protection during stressful situations, in particular Hsp70 expression, might interfere with the acute-phase reaction (circulating cytokines) after a resistance exercise program.[67] Endurance exercise may mediate the anti-inflammatory and antiatrophy effects by many routes, including the upregulation of peroxisome proliferator-activated receptor-γ coactivator (PGC)-1α in muscle, downregulation of Toll-like receptors, and enhanced release of proinflammatory interleukin (IL)-6 by muscles. It has been suggested that mildly elevated expression of PGC-1α in muscle modulates this inflammatory response not only in the muscle itself but also systemically.[68] Downregulation of Toll-like receptors itself modulates inflammation (innate inflammation) in aged subjects and indirectly modulates the sarcopenic process because upregulation of their activity links with the insulin-resistance process.[69] It could be surprising to include IL-6 upregulation as an anti-inflammatory process, but IL-6 inhibits the major inflammation pathway through tumor necrosis factor α (TNF-α) production.[70] For some investigators, an age-related disruption in the intracellular redox balance appears to be a primary causal factor in producing a chronic state of low-grade inflammation, as ROS appear to function as second messengers for TNF-α in skeletal muscle and also activate nuclear factor κB, which itself upregulates IL-6 and TNF-α (see Ref.[71] for review). The effects of exercise training on ROS production could also indirectly modulate the "inflamm-aging."[72] A recent animal study (among nonaged mice) indicated that myostatin could positively alter TNF-α production: modulation of myostatin expression by training could then also be identified as a pathway leading to the anti-inflammatory effect of training.[73]

Effect of Physical Activity on Muscle Denervation in Elderly Subjects

Because mobility-limited older adults exhibited impaired activation of the agonist quadriceps and concomitant deficits in torque and power output whereas healthy subjects did not, it has been suggested that neuromuscular activation deficits may contribute to compromised mobility function in older adults.[74] Aging is characterized by loss of spinal motor neurons due to mechanisms also involved in muscle anabolism and trophicity: apoptosis, reduced IGF-1 signaling, elevated amounts of circulating cytokines, and increased oxidative stress on cells. Therefore, it is of interest to examine whether physical activity could alter the loss of spinal motor neurons.[75] In rats, age-related denervation occurs before myofiber atrophy, and high amounts of neuromuscular activity may delay the onset of age-related denervation and sarcopenia.[76] In humans, strength training appears to be an effective countermeasure in elderly individuals even at a very advanced age (>80 years) by eliciting muscle hypertrophy along with substantial changes in neuromuscular function in the first stages of the plasticity response.[76,77]

Effect of Physical Activity on Muscle and Tendon Architecture in Elderly Subjects

The decrease in muscle volume as a result of aging affects muscle architecture. The decrease in pennation angle and fascicle length during aging has several implications for strength and velocity of contraction.[78] First, a smaller pennation angle leads to a smaller physiologic cross-sectional area (PCSA, which is the ratio of muscle volume to fascicle length, correlated to force production) and also to a simultaneous increase in the force of the muscle fibers exerted on the tendon, proportional to the cosine of the pennation angle[79]; the latter may compensate in part for the smaller PCSA and so for the decrease in force production. The effect of aging on force production is more pronounced for concentric movements (muscle shortening) than for eccentric movements (muscle lengthening). This phenomenon appears to be linked to stiffer muscle structures (in consequence of an accumulation of noncontractile material in the muscle-tendon unit, which offers increased passive stiffness that contributes to musculotendinous eccentric strength) and prolonged myosin cross-bridge cycles of aged muscles.[80,81] Second, muscle fascicle length is routinely reported to be lower in elderly subjects than in young adults. Shorter fascicles (with fewer sarcomeres arranged in series) will generate force over a smaller range of motion and exhibit reduced maximum shortening speed, and they will also generate less force at any given rate of shortening than longer fascicles because their sarcomere shortening rates are higher.[82] Third, protein muscle mass, or contractile tissue, is reduced and as a consequence muscle force is reduced. Fourth, global reduction in muscle force and shortening speed leads to a reduction in muscle power.

Following resistance training, muscle architecture is altered in young, old, and even frail individuals: each of the architectural modifications that occurs with aging and cited above can be partially reversed with training (see Ref.[79] for review). First, resistance exercise training is associated with an increase in pennation angle in old[83] and even frail subjects.[84] An increase in pennation angle is of benefit because more contractile material can be attached to the aponeuroses, as shown by an increase of PCSA, and it generates lateral force transmission. Although this increases the force-generating capacity of the muscle, it can simultaneously reduce the force of the muscle fibers exerted on the tendon, because the cosine of the pennation angle decreases, but the overall force exerted on the tendon remains positive as long as the pennation angle does not exceed 45°.[79] Second, resistance exercise training is associated with an increase in muscle fiber length in old[83] and even frail individuals,[84] which would increase the shortening velocity of the muscle fiber. Third, as discussed in another section, protein muscle mass (contractile tissue) is enhanced by a resistance training program and as a consequence muscle force is increased. Fourth, global increase in muscle force and shortening speed leads to an increase in muscle power.

Aging is also associated with structural modifications of the tendons. In elderly subjects, increased tendon compliance gives a better shortening of the muscle-tendon complex than that measured in a stiff tendon. If one looks closely at the ascending part of the length-tension relation, the greater fascicular shortening during contraction may then contribute to the age-related reduction in specific tension.[78] In a more compliant tendon, a longer time will be needed to stretch the tendon, with the result that less force will be produced over a given time.[9] Two recent topical reviews indicated that the reduction in musculotendinous stiffness in older people can be mitigated by resistance training,[85,86] while a walking training program over 6 months brought about increments in muscle thickness and strength in lower limbs but did not result in any changes in tendon stiffness in the elderly.[87]

Effect of Physical Activity on Muscle Mechanical Excitation-Contraction Coupling in Elderly Subjects

Another factor that may account for the overall effect on the maximum shortening velocity of whole muscle in old age is the impairment of excitation-contraction (E-C) coupling.[88] In fact, the E-C process becomes uncoupled in old age as a consequence of a reduction in T-tubule dihydropyridine receptors and sarcoplasmic reticulum membrane receptors, such as calcium release channels and ryanodine receptors (RyR). This process may result in failure of the transduction of sarcolemmal depolarization into a calcium signal and a mechanical response. Oxidative stress, previously described as a factor that is not specifically age-related but as one that increases during the life span, could also induce qualitative alterations of sarcoplasmic reticulum function,[89] in particular at the RyR level.[90,91] Chronic RyR dysfunction could then be associated with (1) reduced reticular sarcoplasmic calcium release, or (2) chronic calcium leaking with a decreased calcium spike at the E-C coupling time, or (3) an induction of the calcium-dependent apoptotic pathway. Although the effects of regular training and oxidative stress on sarcoplasmic reticulum homeostasis have never been studied in elderly subjects, this countermeasure could have a favorable influence on the E-C process in this population, as it could enhance protein synthesis and reduce oxidative stress (see the preceding sections on this topic).

PHYSICAL ACTIVITY FOR SARCOPENIA: IS THERE AN EVIDENCE-BASED EPIDEMIOLOGIC EFFECT? FROM THE CELL BACK TO HUMAN: IT'S NEVER TOO LATE!

In addition to the beneficial effects, measurable at cell level, of a physical activity program in sarcopenia, the impact of regular physical activity in this context has also been suggested from an epidemiologic viewpoint.

According to an expert panel recently convened for a workshop of The Society for Sarcopenia, Cachexia, and Wasting Disease, exercise (both resistance and aerobic) in combination with adequate protein (leucine-enriched balanced amino acids and possibly creatine) and energy intake is the key component of the prevention and management of sarcopenia (restoring muscle mass and function), whereas adequate protein supplementation alone only slows loss of muscle mass.[92] This assumption is based on evidence-based findings such as those of a recent meta-analysis that aimed to determine the effects of resistance exercise on lean body mass in older men and women, taking exercise regimens and/or age ranges into consideration. Meta-regression revealed that higher volume interventions were associated with significantly greater increases in lean body mass, whereas older individuals experienced less increase.[93,94] The recent prospective study by Park and colleagues[95] also highlighted that after controlling data for age and/or sex, muscle mass increase over 1 year among Japanese subjects aged 65 to 84 years was associated with physical activity, more closely for the legs than for the arms, and for duration of moderate activity (>3 metabolic equivalents [METs]) than for step count. Multivariate-adjusted logistic regressions predicted that seniors who walked at least 7000 to 8000 steps per day and/or spent 15 to 20 minutes per day at an intensity of greater than 3 METs were likely to have a muscle mass above the sarcopenia threshold.

To obtain more robust evidence for the association between sarcopenia and factors such as exercise training, Patel and colleagues[96] suggested that a novel approach combining epidemiologic and basic science characterization of muscle in a well-established birth cohort would allow an integrative investigation of functional and molecular mechanisms underlying life course influences on sarcopenia.

PHYSICAL ACTIVITY FOR SARCOPENIA: HOW TO PRESCRIBE?

Experimental and epidemiologic data have established that physical activity is useful for the primary and tertiary preventions of sarcopenia. It is therefore critical to provide subjects with guidelines to ensure safe and effective practice, just as for drug prescription. Exercise is medicine for chronic disease, and physicians need to prescribe exercise in the same manner as they prescribe drugs.[97] As for any treatment (from oral recommendations to drug prescription), the medical practitioner can first provide patients with guidelines for a physical activity program if he or she is well informed about the rationale and the evidence for this approach; this step of the prescription process is knowledge. Second, the practitioner must be trained to carry out the technical part of the prescription, in particular for physical activity, a therapy implying the patient's active participation. This step of the prescription requires "know-how." Third, still because of the active dimension of the prescription and because any obstacles to physical activity must be identified (personal and environmental obstacles), the practitioner needs to develop self-awareness for social skills. Training is needed to optimize the "know-how" and self-awareness steps. The previous section provided information on the rationale for prescribing physical activity in sarcopenia. The authors now propose a schema to help practitioners standardize their prescription in this field.

When drugs are prescribed, the pharmacologic agent has to be defined (what molecule is recommended for the disease in question?), as well as the dose (appropriate for disease severity and patient characteristics), frequency of drug intake decided (daily or weekly?), duration of treatment, and context of drug administration (does the drug need to be administered in a medical center or not, under the control of a medical or paramedical provider or an instructor, or can the patient take it on his or her own?). When physical activity is considered as a medication, these same domains of health prescription have to be defined. This protocol provides indicators for prescribing a physical activity training program: the prescription needs to define the agent (what kind of physical activity is recommended for the disease in question), the dose to be delivered (appropriate for disease severity and patient characteristics), the frequency of physical activity sessions (whether the dose of physical activity must be taken daily or weekly), and duration and context of the training program (in or outside of a medical center but under the supervision of a health care provider or an instructor, or whether the patient can manage it on his or her own). Both patient and practitioner must be aware that a sedentary lifestyle has more side effects than physical activity.

What Are the Types of Physical Activity?

Individual or collective, indoor or outdoor, with or without a technical support, aquatic or not: these are the defining characteristics of physical activity. The choice made at the time of the prescription will take into account the safety and the efficacy of each type of activity for the disease concerned, the patient's ease of access to the activity, and his or her experience of and pleasure to be gained from it.

How Can the Dose of Physical Activity be Defined?

The dose of physical activity refers to the energy expenditure during the physical activity session. Energy expenditure is itself defined as the product of exercise intensity × exercise duration. The dose of physical activity can thus be altered by modulating exercise intensity and exercise duration.

Defining exercise intensity is a critical step, as it cannot be controlled unequivocally, whereas duration can be timed with a chronometer. Exercise intensity can be defined using subjective indicators such as a scoring scale. For example, the modified Borg Scale (subjective score ranked from 0 to 10) defines moderate intensity as a score from 2 to 4 and high intensity as a score from 5 to 7. The Borg Scale can be used to measure dyspnea, muscle pain, or exercise difficulty.

Exercise intensity can also be defined using objective indicators reflecting the metabolic charge of the exercise. Any muscular contraction needs ATP hydrolysis that releases the energy necessary for sarcomeric actin-myosin cross-bridge cycling. Exercise intensity can be defined as energy output (energy quantity delivered for a time unit, kcal/min for example). The higher the intensity of the exercise, the greater the energy supply and thus the higher the ATP output. In accordance with the kinetic properties of enzymes involved in energy metabolism, phosphagen (stored phosphocreatine and ATP) hydrolysis ensures the maximal ATP production output for muscular contraction but for a short contraction duration, whereas aerobic metabolism ensures minimal ATP production output from fatty acids and carbohydrates (and protein to a small extent) but for a very long contraction duration (lower intensity but more prolonged exercise, defining endurance exercise), and glycolytic metabolism ensures intermediate ATP production output from carbohydrates for an intermediate contraction duration. On a metabolic level, exercise intensity can be defined as low to medium for low to medium levels of energy expenditure corresponding to a low to medium level of recruitment by the aerobic pathway, then as high aerobic intensity and lastly as very high aerobic intensity when the flow of energy expenditure required implies increased glycolytic metabolism and phosphagen, respectively. Whatever the intensity of exercise, all metabolic pathways are recruited at the same time, but the part played by each in the total production of energy varies according to the energy flow required to sustain the muscular exercise imposed.

For aerobic exercises, exercise intensity is defined as the percentage of the maximal oxygen uptake ($V'_{O_{2max}}$; V' is the oxygen consumption output) sustained. For anaerobic exercises, exercise intensity is defined in relation to the maximal force. Assessing and using V'_{O_2} to monitor exercise intensity is not suitable in the whole population because technical support is needed. However, heart rate (HR) can be used as a substitute for V'_{O_2} and is an objective indicator for assessing aerobic exercise intensity. While power increases from rest (R) during a triangular exercise, V'_{O_2} increases linearly to exercise power up to $V'_{O_{2max}}$ and the corresponding maximal (M) aerobic power (AP). While V'_{O_2} increases from R to M-AP, HR rises approximately linearly to V'_{O_2} from R-HR to M-HR. From R to M-AP, V'_{O_2} rises from R-V'_{O_2} to $V'_{O_{2max}}$ and HR rises from R-HR to M-HR, thus defining the heart rate reserve (HRR=M-HR minus R-HR). Because HR and V'_{O_2} are linearly associated with exercise power under the M-AP intensity, the relative intensity of exercise is approximately the same when defined in comparison with M-AP, $V'_{O_{2max}}$, or HRR for an absolute intensity. So for endurance exercises, exercise intensity can also be defined as a percentage of the HRR: low-intensity endurance exercise is defined as 25% to 44% HRR, moderate intensity as 45% to 59% HRR, and high intensity as more than 60% HRR (**Fig. 2**). Defining exercise intensity according to the percentage of HRR is suitable in a clinical population because R-HR can be checked by the physician or the patient in appropriate conditions, while M-HR can be measured at the time of a maximal exercise test or estimated for the corresponding age ($210 - 0.65 \times$ age, for example). Still using cardiac frequency as an exercise intensity indicator, exercise intensity can be

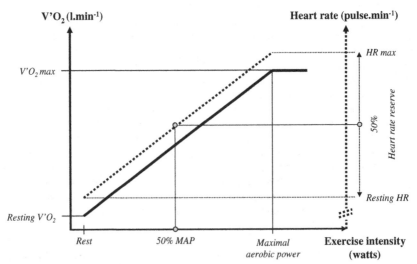

Fig. 2. Definition of endurance exercise: relationship between oxygen consumption (V'_{O_2}), heart rate (HR), and power (P) during an incremental exercise testing procedure. Endurance zone is defined for any exercise intensity below $V'_{O_{2max}}$. Endurance exercise intensity can be derived as a percent of $V'_{O_{2max}}$, or heart rate reserve. MAP, maximal aerobic power.

expressed as a percentage of M-HR: low-intensity endurance exercise is defined as 30% to 49% M-HR, moderate intensity endurance as 50% to 69% M-HR, and high intensity as 70% M-HR. Although it is more direct, this method is less personalized, as it does not take into account the patient's individual resting heart rate, as HRR does. Whatever the cardiac frequency indicator used, exercise intensity can be checked with a cardiofrequency meter.

Finally, intensity can be defined for resistance exercise as a percentage of the maximum repetition test (1-RM, ie, the individual's strength level). Resistance exercise is considered for the purpose of this article from a rehabilitation viewpoint (a slow concentric phase preceded by a slow eccentric phase) and not from a metabolic viewpoint, considering resistance intensity over M-AP.

How Can the Frequency of Physical Activity Sessions Be Defined?

Regularity is a main objective of a training program for patients with chronic diseases. The frequency of physical activity sessions must be defined as days per week. When a daily physical activity dose cannot be administered in a single session, to reach the daily dose two "subdoses" can be taken in the same day, allowing a recovery time between the two. This system is useful for endurance exercise sessions that are longer than resistance sessions, and subdoses should not be less than 10 minutes.

What is the Context of the Training Program?

The context for applying the training program is defined taking into consideration the subject's cognitive capacity, his or her experience of physical activity, motivation, physical capacities, and comorbid diseases, if any. Exercise training can be performed under the control of a medical or a paramedical supervisor, in a center or not, under the supervision of an instructor or without any assistance. Environmental and ecological considerations such as personal resources, access to facilities, and a comfortable setting are central to interventions for the initiation and maintenance of the training program.

Educational Therapy is Central for Exercise Prescription

As a part of any therapeutic prescription, educational therapy is central for exercise prescription and maintenance, whatever the age of the subjects. This method is more central for positive coping strategy therapies such as physical activities. In a recent review, Winett and colleagues[98] emphasized a social cognitive theory–based approach for exercise prescription in older adults. This approach highlights the importance of assisting patients to construct outcome expectancy, self-efficacy, and self-regulation of a physical activity training program. With this aim in mind, a minimal and formal set of personalized recommendations (as proposed below) are needed, while public health policy and programs could be seen as a minimum or "floor" prescription for the general population.

PHYSICAL ACTIVITY FOR SARCOPENIA: WHAT EXERCISE PRESCRIPTION IS RECOMMENDED?

Among the factors affecting a functional response of muscle to exercise training, metabolic and mechanical constraints need to be considered. The level of these constraints differs between endurance and resistance exercise training. Taking into consideration that there are hundreds of muscles of different types in the human body, each of which displays different degrees of atrophy during the aging process, it would be of interest to propose a combination of resistance and endurance training to activate or inhibit some major signaling mechanisms to combat age-related loss and dysfunction of muscle mass. Although combined strength and endurance training regimens can increase endurance performance as well as muscle strength and mass in comparison with strength and endurance training performed separately,[32,99] it has been reported that simultaneous training for both strength and endurance results in a compromised adaptation compared with training with either exercise mode alone.[100] This effect has been variously described as the concurrent training effect or the interference effect,[101] and it highlights a potential bias of combined endurance/strength training studies. This is a nonpaired dose of specific resistance and endurance exercises, as compared with specific resistance or endurance exercise training studies. To better discriminate between the significant exercise stimulatory cues leading to muscular development, a thorough mechanical-biological description of the loading condition is imperative.[102] The key challenges of exercise science for sarcopenia are to best identify the most appropriate muscle-training recommendations for older adults, and to greatly increase the access to safe and effective programs in a variety of settings.

The following section presents the specific effect and value of endurance or resistance exercise in sarcopenic subjects. The authors also address other training methods suggested by recent original published research.

Value of Resistance Training (and Eccentric Exercise) in Sarcopenia

It is resistance exercise that promotes muscle hypertrophy in young and middle-aged individuals (see Ref.[103] for review), and about 2 decades of age-associated loss of strength and muscle mass could be regained in about 2 months of resistance training.[104] The American College of Sport Medicine and the American Heart Association have suggested that training at 70% to 90% of 1-RM (maximal repetition) during 20 to 30 minutes on 2 or more nonconsecutive days per week is the appropriate training intensity to produce gains in muscle size and strength, even in frail elderly subjects.[105,106] It has also been suggested that maintaining the benefits from resistance training in elderly people is possible with as little as one exercise session per week.[107] However, as for young men, myofibrillar protein synthesis is dose-dependent on intensity, and this relationship rises to a plateau at 60% to 90% of 1-RM in older men (70 $\pm$ 5 years), showing anabolic resistance of signaling and myofibrillar protein synthesis to resistance exercise in this population.[20] Moreover, slow movements in resistance exercise are described as creating a high-intensity stimulus while decreasing the chance of injury compared with more rapid movement,[108] but the optimal contraction velocity of muscles is correlated with functional capacity, and power training (force $\times$ velocity) could be a better method of improving velocity and force than concentric training.[82] In summary, recommendation of resistance exercise training to promote muscle hypertrophy and strength in elderly individuals might not be appropriate for sarcopenia. The most appropriate design for a resistance training program to treat or prevent sarcopenia and to prevent physical function and mobility disability in the elderly remains to be defined, therefore more high-quality trials are needed.[109]

As a part of resistance exercise movements, the eccentric contraction mode could also be of specific value in regulating muscle function in elderly subjects. In fact, eccentric strength is better preserved than concentric strength in the elderly: the magnitude of preservation of eccentric strength in older adults ranges from 2% to 48%, with a mean value of 21.6% from all studies, and physical inactivity is cited as a potential factor that could regulate the preservation of eccentric strength.[81] Because low energy cost is coupled to high force production with eccentric exercise and considering this functional reserve of eccentric strength, this intervention may be useful for patients who are otherwise unable to achieve high muscle forces with traditional resistance exercise. This hypothesis has been tested in a few studies: in summary, Raj and colleagues[82] recently proposed that power training and eccentric resistance training could be a better method than traditional resistance training to improve velocity and force and to limit per se muscular functional decline through the life span, but they specify that this should be tested by further targeted studies.

Apart from rehabilitation, the eccentric contraction mode could also be of value in elderly subjects for the assessment of functional capacities through the jumping mechanography method, an integrated approach to evaluation of much of the neuromusculoskeletal system response.[110]

Value of Endurance Training for Sarcopenia

Considering sarcopenia as a lack of muscle mass and muscle strength in older individuals, the authors assumed that resistance was the most specific type of exercise training as a countermeasure. However, it has been suggested that the association between sarcopenia and physical disability could be mediated by decreased cardiopulmonary fitness.[111] Moreover, metabolic diseases that occur in the elderly are altered by endurance capacity. Because an optimal effect on the mechanical and metabolic properties of aged muscle cannot be obtained by a single type of exercise, and considering that endurance training is better than resistance training for developing endurance capacity, it has been suggested that resistance and aerobic training should be combined to combat the global issues of sarcopenia in the elderly population.[112,113] Methods for codifying endurance exercise training have been described in the section "How Can the Dose of Physical Activity be Defined?," and moderate endurance training is recommended in the elderly. However, as for resistance training, the best endurance training regimen for sarcopenic subjects has still not been defined. As an original aerobic training program for sedentary aged people, aerobic interval training (AIT; weekly exercise sessions with 4-minute repetitions at a moderate aerobic intensity alternated with 1-minute repetitions at a sub-high aerobic intensity) could next be considered in sarcopenia. AIT improves aerobic capacity and M-AP in sedentary aged subjects,[114] while a sub-high aerobic intensity repetitions program tends to increase the metabolic stimulus to resistance exercise in an aerobic training program.

Other Training Schemes for Sarcopenia

In recent published studies, Loenneke and colleagues[115] and Fry and colleagues[116] summarized the value of exercise training combined with blood flow restriction to stimulate muscle hypertrophy in older men, and provided original data. Low-intensity occlusion training as low as 20% 1-RM with moderate vascular occlusion results in muscle hypertrophy in older men. Although some of the factors listed here have been identified in acute postexercise sessions (which does not prove their involvement in chronic adaptation of muscle after low-intensity occlusion training), this effect appears to work through a variety of mechanisms such as metabolic accumulation (stimulating a subsequent increase in anabolic growth factors), fast-twitch fiber recruitment, increased protein synthesis through the mTOR pathway, and modulation of ribosomal activity. Hsps, Nitric oxide synthase 1, and myostatin have also been shown to be affected by an occlusion stimulus.

The effect of vibration training on skeletal muscle has also been studied in the elderly. In an intervention study without a control group among elderly women and men (65–85 years of age), Pietrangelo and colleagues[117] observed that vibration training could lead to enhanced maximal isometric strength with cellular and molecular adaptations, which include chronic changes in pathways related with energy metabolism, sarcomere protein balance, and oxidative stress response, but no increase in fiber or muscle. The usefulness of vibration training for sarcopenia rehabilitation needs to be determined through further standardized studies.[118]

SUMMARY

Evidence exists that muscle weakness, reduction in muscle mass, and reduction in physical activity occur during the life span, and lead to sarcopenia and disability in some older subjects. Evidence also exists that physical activity, which is a modifiable lifestyle behavior, can partially reverse age-associated skeletal muscle dysfunction. The links between a disease and a countermeasure, and the behavioral and environmental obstacles to access to this countermeasure for the practitioner and the patient, must be identified to optimize its prescription. While further studies are needed to identify the best qualitative and quantitative training regimen for sarcopenic subjects, the authors also propose the encouragement of "double-target" training: practitioners should be encouraged to "train" their knowledge and skill in exercise therapy through exercise prescription according to the present recommendations in order to provide good medical and practical support to sarcopenic patients for their training program.

REFERENCES

1. Muscaritoli M, Anker SD, Argiles J, et al. Consensus definition of sarcopenia, cachexia and pre-cachexia: joint document elaborated by Special Interest Groups (SIG) "cachexia-anorexia in chronic wasting diseases" and "nutrition in geriatrics". Clin Nutr 2010;29:154.
2. Cruz-Jentoft AJ, Baeyens JP, Bauer JM, et al. Sarcopenia: European consensus on definition and diagnosis: Report of the European Working Group on Sarcopenia in Older People. Age Ageing 2010;39:412.
3. Visser M, Newman AB, Nevitt MC, et al. Reexamining the sarcopenia hypothesis. Muscle mass versus muscle strength. Health, Aging, and Body Composition Study Research Group. Ann N Y Acad Sci 2000;904:456.
4. D'Antona G, Pellegrino MA, Carlizzi CN, et al. Deterioration of contractile properties of muscle fibres in elderly subjects is modulated by the level of physical activity. Eur J Appl Physiol 2007;100:603.
5. Degens H, Alway SE. Control of muscle size during disuse, disease, and aging. Int J Sports Med 2006;27:94.
6. Kortebein P, Ferrando A, Lombeida J, et al. Effect of 10 days of bed rest on skeletal muscle in healthy older adults. JAMA 2007;297:1772.
7. Lee JS, Auyeung TW, Kwok T, et al. Associated factors and health impact of sarcopenia in older Chinese men and women: a cross-sectional study. Gerontology 2007;53:404.
8. Nair KS. Aging muscle. Am J Clin Nutr 2005;81:953.
9. Reeves ND, Narici MV, Maganaris CN. Myotendinous plasticity to ageing and resistance exercise in humans. Exp Physiol 2006;91:483.
10. Bamman MM, Ragan RC, Kim JS, et al. Myogenic protein expression before and after resistance loading in 26- and 64-yr-old men and women. J Appl Physiol 2004;97:1329.
11. Kim JS, Kosek DJ, Petrella JK, et al. Resting and load-induced levels of myogenic gene transcripts differ between older adults with demonstrable sarcopenia and young men and women. J Appl Physiol 2005;99:2149.

12. Raue U, Slivka D, Jemiolo B, et al. Myogenic gene expression at rest and after a bout of resistance exercise in young (18-30 yr) and old (80-89 yr) women. J Appl Physiol 2006;101:53.
13. Edstrom E, Ulfhake B. Sarcopenia is not due to lack of regenerative drive in senescent skeletal muscle. Aging Cell 2005;4:65.
14. Frontera WR, Reid KF, Phillips EM, et al. Muscle fiber size and function in elderly humans: a longitudinal study. J Appl Physiol 2008;105:637.
15. Buford TW, Anton SD, Judge AR, et al. Models of accelerated sarcopenia: Critical pieces for solving the puzzle of age-related muscle atrophy. Ageing Res Rev 2010;9(4):369–83.
16. Wang X, Proud CG. The mTOR pathway in the control of protein synthesis. Physiology (Bethesda) 2006;21:362.
17. Rivas DA, Lessard SJ, Coffey VG. mTOR function in skeletal muscle: a focal point for overnutrition and exercise. Appl Physiol Nutr Metab 2009;34:807.
18. Hulmi JJ, Tannerstedt J, Selanne H, et al. Resistance exercise with whey protein ingestion affects mTOR signaling pathway and myostatin in men. J Appl Physiol 2009;106:1720.
19. Drummond MJ, Dreyer HC, Pennings B, et al. Skeletal muscle protein anabolic response to resistance exercise and essential amino acids is delayed with aging. J Appl Physiol 2008;104:1452.
20. Kumar V, Selby A, Rankin D, et al. Age-related differences in the dose-response relationship of muscle protein synthesis to resistance exercise in young and old men. J Physiol 2009;587:211.
21. Yarasheski KE, Bhasin S, Sinha-Hikim I, et al. Serum myostatin-immunoreactive protein is increased in 60-92 year old women and men with muscle wasting. J Nutr Health Aging 2002;6:343.
22. Kosek DJ, Kim JS, Petrella JK, et al. Efficacy of 3 days/wk resistance training on myofiber hypertrophy and myogenic mechanisms in young vs. older adults. J Appl Physiol 2006;101:531.
23. Snijders T, Verdijk LB, van Loon LJ. The impact of sarcopenia and exercise training on skeletal muscle satellite cells. Ageing Res Rev 2009;8:328.
24. Vettor R, Milan G, Franzin C, et al. The origin of intermuscular adipose tissue and its pathophysiological implications. Am J Physiol Endocrinol Metab 2009;297:E987-8.
25. Koopman R, van Loon LJ. Aging, exercise, and muscle protein metabolism. J Appl Physiol 2009;106:2040.
26. Sakuma K, Yamaguchi A. Molecular mechanisms in aging and current strategies to counteract sarcopenia. Curr Aging Sci 2010;3:90.
27. Alway SE, Siu PM. Nuclear apoptosis contributes to sarcopenia. Exerc Sport Sci Rev 2008;36:51.
28. Song W, Kwak HB, Lawler JM. Exercise training attenuates age-induced changes in apoptotic signaling in rat skeletal muscle. Antioxid Redox Signal 2006;8:517.
29. Wohlgemuth SE, Seo AY, Marzetti E, et al. Skeletal muscle autophagy and apoptosis during aging: effects of calorie restriction and life-long exercise. Exp Gerontol 2010;45:138.
30. Wilkes EA, Selby AL, Atherton PJ, et al. Blunting of insulin inhibition of proteolysis in legs of older subjects may contribute to age-related sarcopenia. Am J Clin Nutr 2009;90:1343.
31. Lanza IR, Short DK, Short KR, et al. Endurance exercise as a countermeasure for aging. Diabetes 2008;57:2933.

32. Ahtiainen JP, Hulmi JJ, Kraemer WJ, et al. Strength, endurance or combined training elicit diverse skeletal muscle myosin heavy chain isoform proportion but unaltered androgen receptor concentration in older men. Int J Sports Med 2009;30:879.

33. Kraemer WJ, Ratamess NA. Hormonal responses and adaptations to resistance exercise and training. Sports Med 2005;35:339.

34. Ratamess NA, Kraemer WJ, Volek JS, et al. Androgen receptor content following heavy resistance exercise in men. J Steroid Biochem Mol Biol 2005;93:35.

35. Spiering BA, Kraemer WJ, Vingren JL, et al. Elevated endogenous testosterone concentrations potentiate muscle androgen receptor responses to resistance exercise. J Steroid Biochem Mol Biol 2009;114:195.

36. Rahman F, Christian HC. Non-classical actions of testosterone: an update. Trends Endocrinol Metab 2007;18:371.

37. Narici MV, Maffulli N. Sarcopenia: characteristics, mechanisms and functional significance. Br Med Bull 2010;95:139.

38. Rolland Y, Czerwinski S, Abellan Van Kan G, et al. Sarcopenia: its assessment, etiology, pathogenesis, consequences and future perspectives. J Nutr Health Aging 2008;12:433.

39. Sipila S, Taaffe DR, Cheng S, et al. Effects of hormone replacement therapy and high-impact physical exercise on skeletal muscle in post-menopausal women: a randomized placebo-controlled study. Clin Sci (Lond) 2001;101:147.

40. Singh MA, Ding W, Manfredi TJ, et al. Insulin-like growth factor I in skeletal muscle after weight-lifting exercise in frail elders. Am J Physiol 1999;277:E135.

41. Hameed M, Lange KH, Andersen JL, et al. The effect of recombinant human growth hormone and resistance training on IGF-I mRNA expression in the muscles of elderly men. J Physiol 2004;555:231.

42. Hand BD, Kostek MC, Ferrell RE, et al. Influence of promoter region variants of insulin-like growth factor pathway genes on the strength-training response of muscle phenotypes in older adults. J Appl Physiol 2007;103:1678.

43. Karagounis LG, Hawley JA. Skeletal muscle: increasing the size of the locomotor cell. Int J Biochem Cell Biol 2010;42:1376.

44. Waters DL, Brooks WM, Qualls CR, et al. Skeletal muscle mitochondrial function and lean body mass in healthy exercising elderly. Mech Ageing Dev 2003; 124:301.

45. Melov S, Tarnopolsky MA, Beckman K, et al. Resistance exercise reverses aging in human skeletal muscle. PLoS One 2007;2:e465.

46. Lanza IR, Nair KS. Muscle mitochondrial changes with aging and exercise. Am J Clin Nutr 2009;89:467S.

47. Safdar A, Hamadeh MJ, Kaczor JJ, et al. Aberrant mitochondrial homeostasis in the skeletal muscle of sedentary older adults. PLoS One 2010;5:e10778.

48. McCully KK, Posner JD. The application of blood flow measurements to the study of aging muscle. J Gerontol A Biol Sci Med Sci 1995;50(Spec No):130.

49. Rogers MA, Evans WJ. Changes in skeletal muscle with aging: effects of exercise training. Exerc Sport Sci Rev 1993;21:65.

50. Ochi M, Kohara K, Tabara Y, et al. Arterial stiffness is associated with low thigh muscle mass in middle-aged to elderly men. Atherosclerosis 2010;212:327.

51. Payne GW. Effect of inflammation on the aging microcirculation: impact on skeletal muscle blood flow control. Microcirculation 2006;13:343.

52. Chow LS, Greenlund LJ, Asmann YW, et al. Impact of endurance training on murine spontaneous activity, muscle mitochondrial DNA abundance, gene transcripts, and function. J Appl Physiol 2007;102:1078.

53. Cartee GD. Aging skeletal muscle: response to exercise. Exerc Sport Sci Rev 1994;22:91.
54. Brooks GA, Mercier J. Balance of carbohydrate and lipid utilization during exercise: the "crossover" concept. J Appl Physiol 1994;76:2253.
55. Hue L, Taegtmeyer H. The Randle cycle revisited: a new head for an old hat. Am J Physiol Endocrinol Metab 2009;297:E578.
56. Crentsil V. Mechanistic contribution of carnitine deficiency to geriatric frailty. Ageing Res Rev 2010;9:265.
57. Thomson DM, Brown JD, Fillmore N, et al. AMP-activated protein kinase response to contractions and treatment with the AMPK activator AICAR in young adult and old skeletal muscle. J Physiol 2009;587:2077.
58. Schrauwen P, Russell AP, Moonen-Kornips E, et al. Effect of 2 weeks of endurance training on uncoupling protein 3 content in untrained human subjects. Acta Physiol Scand 2005;183:273.
59. Gosker HR, Schrauwen P, Broekhuizen R, et al. Exercise training restores uncoupling protein-3 content in limb muscles of patients with chronic obstructive pulmonary disease. Am J Physiol Endocrinol Metab 2006;290:E976.
60. Combaret L, Dardevet D, Bechet D, et al. Skeletal muscle proteolysis in aging. Curr Opin Clin Nutr Metab Care 2009;12:37.
61. Fulle S, Di Donna S, Puglielli C, et al. Age-dependent imbalance of the antioxidative system in human satellite cells. Exp Gerontol 2005;40:189.
62. Jang YC, Lustgarten MS, Liu Y, et al. Increased superoxide in vivo accelerates age-associated muscle atrophy through mitochondrial dysfunction and neuromuscular junction degeneration. FASEB J 2010;24:1376.
63. Semba RD, Ferrucci L, Sun K, et al. Oxidative stress and severe walking disability among older women. Am J Med 2007;120:1084.
64. Ristow M, Zarse K. How increased oxidative stress promotes longevity and metabolic health: the concept of mitochondrial hormesis (mitohormesis). Exp Gerontol 2010;45:410.
65. Ji LL. Exercise-induced modulation of antioxidant defense. Ann N Y Acad Sci 2002;959:82.
66. Buford TW, Cooke MB, Willoughby DS. Resistance exercise-induced changes of inflammatory gene expression within human skeletal muscle. Eur J Appl Physiol 2009;107:463.
67. Bautmans I, Njemini R, Vasseur S, et al. Biochemical changes in response to intensive resistance exercise training in the elderly. Gerontology 2005;51:253.
68. Wenz T, Rossi SG, Rotundo RL, et al. Increased muscle PGC-1alpha expression protects from sarcopenia and metabolic disease during aging. Proc Natl Acad Sci U S A 2009;106:20405.
69. Frisard MI, McMillan RP, Marchand J, et al. Toll-like receptor 4 modulates skeletal muscle substrate metabolism. Am J Physiol Endocrinol Metab 2010;298:E988.
70. Petersen AM, Pedersen BK. The anti-inflammatory effect of exercise. J Appl Physiol 2005;98:1154.
71. Chung HY, Cesari M, Anton S, et al. Molecular inflammation: underpinnings of aging and age-related diseases. Ageing Res Rev 2009;8:18.
72. Shaw AC, Joshi S, Greenwood H, et al. Aging of the innate immune system. Curr Opin Immunol 2010;22:507.
73. Wilkes JJ, Lloyd DJ, Gekakis N. Loss-of-function mutation in myostatin reduces tumor necrosis factor alpha production and protects liver against obesity-induced insulin resistance. Diabetes 2009;58:1133.

74. Clark DJ, Patten C, Reid KF, et al. Impaired voluntary neuromuscular activation limits muscle power in mobility-limited older adults. J Gerontol A Biol Sci Med Sci 2010;65:495.

75. Aagaard P, Suetta C, Caserotti P, et al. Role of the nervous system in sarcopenia and muscle atrophy with aging: strength training as a countermeasure. Scand J Med Sci Sports 2010;20:49.

76. Deschenes MR, Roby MA, Eason MK, et al. Remodeling of the neuromuscular junction precedes sarcopenia related alterations in myofibers. Exp Gerontol 2010;45:389.

77. Frontera WR, Hughes VA, Krivickas LS, et al. Strength training in older women: early and late changes in whole muscle and single cells. Muscle Nerve 2003; 28:601.

78. Morse CI, Thom JM, Reeves ND, et al. In vivo physiological cross-sectional area and specific force are reduced in the gastrocnemius of elderly men. J Appl Physiol 2005;99:1050.

79. Degens H, Erskine RM, Morse CI. Disproportionate changes in skeletal muscle strength and size with resistance training and ageing. J Musculoskelet Neuronal Interact 2009;9:123.

80. Vandervoort AA. Aging of the human neuromuscular system. Muscle Nerve 2002;25:17.

81. Roig M, Macintyre DL, Eng JJ, et al. Preservation of eccentric strength in older adults: evidence, mechanisms and implications for training and rehabilitation. Exp Gerontol 2010;45:400.

82. Raj IS, Bird SR, Shield AJ. Aging and the force-velocity relationship of muscles. Exp Gerontol 2010;45:81.

83. Reeves ND, Narici MV, Maganaris CN. In vivo human muscle structure and function: adaptations to resistance training in old age. Exp Physiol 2004;89:675.

84. Suetta C, Andersen JL, Dalgas U, et al. Resistance training induces qualitative changes in muscle morphology, muscle architecture, and muscle function in elderly postoperative patients. J Appl Physiol 2008;105:180.

85. Magnusson SP, Narici MV, Maganaris CN, et al. Human tendon behaviour and adaptation, in vivo. J Physiol 2008;586:71.

86. Narici MV, Maffulli N, Maganaris CN. Ageing of human muscles and tendons. Disabil Rehabil 2008;30:1548.

87. Kubo K, Ishida Y, Suzuki S, et al. Effects of 6 months of walking training on lower limb muscle and tendon in elderly. Scand J Med Sci Sports 2008;18:31.

88. Delbono O. Regulation of excitation contraction coupling by insulin-like growth factor-1 in aging skeletal muscle. J Nutr Health Aging 2000;4:162.

89. Galbes O, Bourret A, Nouette-Gaulain K, et al. N-acetylcysteine protects against bupivacaine-induced myotoxicity caused by oxidative and sarcoplasmic reticulum stress in human skeletal myotubes. Anesthesiology 2010;113:560.

90. Arbogast S, Beuvin M, Fraysse B, et al. Oxidative stress in SEPN1-related myopathy: from pathophysiology to treatment. Ann Neurol 2009;65:677.

91. Terentyev D, Gyorke I, Belevych AE, et al. Redox modification of ryanodine receptors contributes to sarcoplasmic reticulum Ca^{2+} leak in chronic heart failure. Circ Res 2008;103:1466.

92. Morley JE, Argiles JM, Evans WJ, et al. Nutritional recommendations for the management of sarcopenia. J Am Med Dir Assoc 2010;11:391.

93. Peterson MD, Sen A, Gordon PM. Influence of resistance exercise on lean body mass in aging adults: a meta-analysis. Med Sci Sports Exerc 2011;43(2): 249–58.

94. Peterson MD, Rhea MR, Sen A, et al. Resistance exercise for muscular strength in older adults: a meta-analysis. Ageing Res Rev 2010;9:226.
95. Park H, Park S, Shephard RJ, et al. Yearlong physical activity and sarcopenia in older adults: the Nakanojo Study. Eur J Appl Physiol 2010;109:953.
96. Patel HP, Syddall HE, Martin HJ, et al. Hertfordshire sarcopenia study: design and methods. BMC Geriatr 2010;10:43.
97. Sallis RE. Exercise is medicine and physicians need to prescribe it! Br J Sports Med 2009;43:3.
98. Winett RA, Williams DM, Davy BM. Initiating and maintaining resistance training in older adults: a social cognitive theory-based approach. Br J Sports Med 2009;43:114.
99. Sillanpaa E, Hakkinen A, Nyman K, et al. Body composition and fitness during strength and/or endurance training in older men. Med Sci Sports Exerc 2008; 40:950.
100. Hawley JA. Molecular responses to strength and endurance training: are they incompatible? Appl Physiol Nutr Metab 2009;34:355.
101. Nader GA. Concurrent strength and endurance training: from molecules to man. Med Sci Sports Exerc 1965;38:2006.
102. Toigo M, Boutellier U. New fundamental resistance exercise determinants of molecular and cellular muscle adaptations. Eur J Appl Physiol 2006;97:643.
103. Meng SJ, Yu LJ. Oxidative stress, molecular inflammation and sarcopenia. Int J Mol Sci 2010;11:1509.
104. Hurley BF, Roth SM. Strength training in the elderly: effects on risk factors for age-related diseases. Sports Med 2000;30:249.
105. Borst SE. Interventions for sarcopenia and muscle weakness in older people. Age Ageing 2004;33:548.
106. Nelson ME, Rejeski WJ, Blair SN, et al. Physical activity and public health in older adults: recommendation from the American College of Sports Medicine and the American Heart Association. Med Sci Sports Exerc 2007;39:1435.
107. Taaffe DR, Duret C, Wheeler S, et al. Once-weekly resistance exercise improves muscle strength and neuromuscular performance in older adults. J Am Geriatr Soc 1999;47:1208.
108. Winett RA, Carpinelli RN. Potential health-related benefits of resistance training. Prev Med 2001;33:503.
109. Chin MJ, van Uffelen JG, Riphagen I, et al. The functional effects of physical exercise training in frail older people: a systematic review. Sports Med 2008; 38:781.
110. Buehring B, Krueger D, Binkley N. Jumping mechanography: a potential tool for sarcopenia evaluation in older individuals. J Clin Densitom 2010;13:283.
111. Chien MY, Kuo HK, Wu YT. Sarcopenia, cardiopulmonary fitness, and physical disability in community-dwelling elderly people. Phys Ther 2010;90:1277.
112. Harber MP, Konopka AR, Douglass MD, et al. Aerobic exercise training improves whole muscle and single myofiber size and function in older women. Am J Physiol Regul Integr Comp Physiol 2009;297:R1452.
113. Hunter GR, McCarthy JP, Bamman MM. Effects of resistance training on older adults. Sports Med 2004;34:329.
114. Lepretre PM, Vogel T, Brechat PH, et al. Impact of a short-term aerobic interval training on maximal exercise in sedentary aged subjects. Int J Clin Pract 2009; 63:1472.
115. Loenneke JP, Wilson GJ, Wilson JM. A mechanistic approach to blood flow occlusion. Int J Sports Med 2010;31:1.

116. Fry CS, Glynn EL, Drummond MJ, et al. Blood flow restriction exercise stimulates mTORC1 signaling and muscle protein synthesis in older men. J Appl Physiol 2010;108:1199.

117. Pietrangelo T, Mancinelli R, Toniolo L, et al. Effects of local vibrations on skeletal muscle trophism in elderly people: mechanical, cellular, and molecular events. Int J Mol Med 2009;24:503.

118. Santin-Medeiros F, Garatachea Vallejo N. Musculoskeletal effects of vibration training in the elderly. Rev Esp Geriatr Gerontol 2010;45(5):281–4 [in Spanish].

Clinical Trials on Sarcopenia: Methodological Issues Regarding Phase 3 Trials

Gabor Abellan van Kan, MD[a,b,*],
Wm. Cameron Chumlea, MD, PhD[c],
Sophie Gillette-Guyonet, PhD[a,b], Mathieu Houles, MD[a],
Charlotte Dupuy, MSPT[a,b], Yves Rolland, MD, PhD[a,b],
Bruno Vellas, MD, PhD[a,b]

KEYWORDS

• Sarcopenia • Older adults • Clinical trial • Methodology

Sarcopenia was initially defined as an age-related loss of muscle mass[1] but this definition and the biological and clinical concept of sarcopenia have dramatically evolved to try to address a broader perspective on this important part of the aging process. However, current research on the plausible mechanistic pathways leading to sarcopenia and the functional consequences of sarcopenia are hampered by a lack of a consensus definition and a standardized assessment methodology.[2,3] This issue is currently addressed by numerous international scientific and clinical groups with limited success.[4] The lack of a clear definition of sarcopenia and an assessment methodology results in a variation in the reported prevalence across available representative epidemiologic cohorts of between 8% and 40%.[2] This broad range in prevalence and the absence of consensus criteria make the performance and outcomes of phase 3 clinical trials challenging. A large variability in the target population, if uncontrolled, increases the uncertainty in possible drug effects by inflating the confidence intervals, and attempts to control the variability by using

For this work, Dr Chumlea, was supported in part by grant HD-12252 from the National Institutes of Health, Bethesda, MD, USA.

[a] Gérontopôle, Department of Geriatric Medicine, Toulouse University Hospital, 170, avenue de Casselardit, 31059 Toulouse, Cedex 9, France
[b] INSERM, Unit 1027, University Toulouse-III, Avenue Jules Guesde, 31059 Toulouse, France
[c] Lifespan Health Research Center, Department of Community Health, Boonshoft School of Medicine, Wright State University, 3640 Colonel Glenn Highway, Dayton, OH 45435, USA
* Corresponding author. Gérontopôle, Department of Geriatric Medicine, Toulouse University Hospital, 170, avenue de Casselardit, 31059 Toulouse, cedex 9, France.
E-mail address: abellan-van-kan-g@chu-toulouse.fr

Clin Geriatr Med 27 (2011) 471–482
doi:10.1016/j.cger.2011.03.010   **geriatric.theclinics.com**
0749-0690/11/$ – see front matter © 2011 Elsevier Inc. All rights reserved.

a homogeneous less-representative study population reduces the generalizability of the drug effects, thus questioning the clinical efficacy of these trials. It is noteworthy to state that the challenges to conduct phase 3 trials in the elderly should not offset the opportunities for the development of new strategies to counteract sarcopenia and prevent late-life disability.

This article comprehensively reviews the methodological issues of conducting phase 3 clinical trials for sarcopenia. The current sarcopenia definition, body composition assessment, target population, end points, the need of biologic markers, and the design of phase 3 trials are further developed throughout this article.

METHODOLOGY

A PubMed search with the MeSH terms, sarcopenia (all subheadings): clinical trial, phase 3, body composition, sarcopenia-aged-80 and over-frail elderly, was performed to retrieve relevant articles published from 2008 through 2010. Abstracts of the articles were reviewed, and selected publications were consulted in full. The reference lists of the selected articles were also pearled for supportive relevant literature, and the investigators provided additional articles of interest to obtain a more comprehensive review of the literature.

DEFINING PHASE 3 CLINICAL TRIALS

Clinical trials are used to assess the performance and safety of new pharmaceutical agents, and they are classified into 4 phases, 1 to 4. **Table 1** summarizes the main features of each of the phases. Before approval by government regulatory authorities and commercialization, a new drug is tested in separate trials in each of the 3 initial phases. Phase 4 is the postmarketing phase with intensive safety surveillance after a drug is commercially available. Phase 3 clinical trials are randomized controlled trials on large patient groups aimed at providing a definitive assessment of efficacy in clinical use. Because of their size and long duration, phase 3 trials are expensive, time consuming, and difficult to design and run.

DEFINITION OF SARCOPENIA

Since its first description, various definitions of sarcopenia have appeared as the knowledge and understanding of the aging process have increased. During this time, improved techniques to assess body composition and the availability of large

Table 1
Phases of clinical trials during drug development

Phase	Subjects	Main End Points
Phase 1	Trial in a small group of healthy volunteers	Safety and tolerability Pharmacokinetics and pharmacodynamics
Phase 2	Trial in a larger group of healthy volunteers or patients	2A: antidisease activity and dose assessment 2B: efficacy of the drug
Phase 3	Randomized controlled trial in a large group of patients	Assessment of the efficacy of a drug Approval to market the drug
Phase 4	Trial in drug-prescribed patients Postmarketing trial	Safety surveillance (pharmacovigilance)

representative epidemiologic data sets have modified the initial simple concept of a decrease in the muscle mass. Despite these enhancements in basic and clinical knowledge and technology, a consensus operational definition of sarcopenia applicable across racial groups/ethnic groups/populations has not developed.[2] The current definitions of sarcopenia add a loss in strength and a decline in function to the loss of muscle mass,[4–6] but it is unclear whether muscle weakness results from the loss of muscle mass or from a qualitative histologic impairment of muscle tissue. Muscle mass declines at a rate of 1% to 2% per year after 50 years of age, but strength declines at 1.5% per year and is as much as 3% per year after the age of 60 years. Even if this decline in strength is higher in sedentary individuals, and twice as high in men than in women, less than 5% of the variance in the age-related decline in strength is explained by concurrent changes in muscle mass.[7] Despite the actual controversies, the available data for sarcopenia are sufficient to designate that the decline in muscle mass is a primary determinant of the disabling process associated with sarcopenia. It could be less relevant than muscle strength or physical performance in predicting clinical events, but loss of lean mass is associated with major biologic and clinical outcomes.[3]

Most current definitions of sarcopenia are based on a cut point for low total or appendicular lean mass, and some have started to include measures of strength or physical performance.[8,9] This inclusion is because of recent knowledge that numerous mechanisms, beyond muscle mass, underlie the cause for muscle weakness in the elderly. Impairments in the muscular and/or nervous systems (with the possibility that cognitive decline acts as a determinant), physical inactivity, and chronic undernutrition, along with hormonal declines and immunologic changes in the physiology of older adults, contribute to this broader view of sarcopenia.[4,9] A recent proposed diagnosis of sarcopenia required the documentation of low muscle mass and the presence of low strength as measured by grip strength or low physical performance as measured by gait speed.[4] Walking requires muscle mass, function, and strength. Grip strength is a useful surrogate for total strength in young adults but can be compromised by arthritis and functional use in the hands. Gait speed, at the usual pace and over a short distance, is a reliable, valid, and quick physical performance assessment tool and a major predictor of adverse health outcomes with specific cut points for many diseases.[5] These characteristics indicate that gait speed is potentially the main screening tool for the presence of sarcopenia along with low muscle mass in the elderly.[4]

TARGET POPULATIONS

The possible target populations should have a sarcopenia risk profile to provide the required clinical end points and optimize the statistical power to detect a meaningful difference between the intervention and the control group, to diminish the sample size, and to decrease the duration of the trial.[10] However, the absence of a consensus definition of sarcopenia makes it difficult to determine the best target population. A broad definition of sarcopenia leads to a target population with high variability in which it is difficult to detect meaningful differences but it is easy to generalize. A restricted definition of sarcopenia leads to a target population with low variability but a low capacity of generalization of findings. In addition, the overall goal of the trial needs to be considered. For example, a primary preventive trial would require a presarcopenia stage target population with a risk profile without presenting sarcopenia. The presarcopenia stage has been recently conceptualized by low muscle mass without an effect on strength or physical performance.[4] **Table 2** summarizes the new concepts of presarcopenia, sarcopenia, and severe sarcopenia. In sarcopenia preventive trials, the

Parameter Assessed	Proposed Measurement	Presarcopenia	Sarcopenia	Severe Sarcopenia
Table 2 Conceptual stages of sarcopenia				
Lean Mass	DXA	Decreased	Decreased	Decreased
Strength Physical performance	Hand grip Gait speed	Normal	Decreased strength or Decreased physical performance	Decreased strength and Decreased physical performance

Abbreviation: DXA, dual-energy x-ray absorptiometry.
Data from Cruz-Jentoft A, Baeyens JP, Bauer J, et al. Sarcopenia: European consensus on definition and diagnosis: report of the European working group on sarcopenia in older people. Age Ageing 2010;39:414.

variability can be large if inclusion is based solely on muscle mass assessment and large populations need to be included to power the study. If an intervention yields positive results (delays the onset of functional impairment or forces decline in the presence of low muscle mass), it could be generalized to the whole aging population. However, for clinical trials assessing an intervention, not only muscle impairment but also a decline in strength or physical performance (at a sarcopenic or severe sarcopenic stage) needs to be present. The target population must therefore be much more selective to exclude not only sarcopenic patients but also disabled older adults. Primary preventive trials should be conducted in autonomous, community-dwelling older adults who present with few disabilities, and so, strength measurements and physical performance assessment should not be impaired. Intervention trials can be conducted not only in community-dwelling autonomous older adults but also in specific communities presenting some degree of disability. The enrollment of specific populations such as institutionalized or hospitalized older adults (because of acute diseases or surgery or because of programmed elective surgery) depends on the goal of the study. If disability is present, the assessment tools need to be adapted to the degree of dependency of the target population. Depending on the study population, slight to severe impairments should be observed in strength, physical performance, and muscle mass.

Another major challenge in selecting the target population is the presence of coexisting conditions with a wide spectrum of potential confounders able to influence skeletal muscle. Comorbidities need to be standardized to obtain a clear baseline with no confounders, but this standardization depends on the age range of the target group and increasing difficulty in the oldest age groups. Nutritional status needs to be assessed, and malnutrition should probably be considered as an exclusion criterion in the same way as the presence of severe functional impairment. The lack of careful characterization can explain why many clinical trials on sarcopenia, especially those that tested pharmacologic agents, have been disappointing.[11]

Clearly, the first aim is to define sarcopenia (muscle mass and/or muscle weakness) depending on the overall goal of the trial, measure all possible confounders, and then decide how to account for them using design and analytic strategies. Two possible strategies, to account for confounders, are possible. The first is to state restrictive inclusion-exclusion criteria so that a homogeneous population is included in the trial. The second is to perform stratification based on previous identified confounders when analyzing the trial data. This strategy needs to be planned during the design of the study because the sample size needs to be increased.

Finally, the sarcopenia risk profile could be increased by increasing the age of the trial participants. The main manifestations of the age-related muscle loss are evident at old age; therefore, in order to evaluate whether an intervention is beneficial in the delay of sarcopenia onset or the treatment of sarcopenia, sarcopenia-related impairments must be present (for an intervention trial) or appear over a short period (for a prevention trial). Taking into account the prevalence of sarcopenia in community-dwelling older adults (about 10% in older adults aged 60–70 years and about 30% in those older than 80 years), the target population could be those aged 70 years or older.[12] In a younger population, sarcopenia would be hard to identify and too many participants will need to be screened; even more, the onset of sarcopenia-related impairments will be expected to develop over a longer period so that the duration of follow-up of this sample will be an issue.

SARCOPENIA ASSESSMENT: SKELETAL MUSCLE MASS

A wide range of techniques are available to assess muscle mass.[13] The most commonly used, low cost, and accessible method to assess skeletal muscle mass is dual-energy x-ray absorptiometry (DXA). The accuracy of DXA for assessing muscle mass in people of different age groups and in some pathologic conditions may vary. DXA overestimates muscle mass because it does not differentiate between water and bone-free lean tissue. Despite these limitations, DXA provides valid estimates of appendicular skeletal muscle mass, and skeletal muscle measures with DXA are associated with prevalent and incident physical disability. Bioelectric impedance analysis is an inexpensive and easy-to-assess methodology but has limited accuracy and validity and is not broadly recommended for use among older adults. Similarly, anthropometric measures are not recommended for the assessment of skeletal muscle mass in the elderly.[4] Magnetic resonance imaging (MRI) and computed tomography (CT) are considered the gold standard and the most accurate imaging methods to assess muscle mass, muscle cross-sectional area, and muscle quality as determined by muscle density and intramuscular fat infiltration. However, the high cost and operational complexity limit their use in large clinical trials. MRI and CT also assess adipose tissue, which is directly associated with intramuscular fat infiltrates, which in turn may impair muscle function and strength.[14]

Skeletal muscle mass assessment should be performed by DXA in trials in which large samples are needed, such as preventive trials, when initially assessing the muscle mass as a case-finding tool; when lean, fat, and bone tissues need to be assessed at the same time; or when repeated measurements are needed (because DXA exposes to minimum radiation). MRI or CT should be reserved for more-specific trials during drug development in smaller samples but in which muscle density and fat infiltration is an issue and mainly for proof of concept. Reducing fat infiltration or increasing muscle density could result in muscle quality improvement without increases in muscle mass (therefore not detected by DXA) and therefore prove efficacy of certain interventions.

SARCOPENIA ASSESSMENT: STRENGTH AND PHYSICAL PERFORMANCE

Skeletal muscle strength is an important component for the assessment of sarcopenia and muscle quality. Several measurement methods are available, including simple dynamometers to measure isometric strength of the hand and forearm and the complex isokinetic strength measures of power and torque of the legs. Muscle strength measures of various body compartments are correlated. Grip strength measured with a hand dynamometer is a reasonable surrogate measure of skeletal muscle strength in the lower extremities,[13] and it is a clinical marker of adverse outcomes, showing a predictive value for mortality similar to that of quadriceps strength.[15,16] However, grip strength can be difficult to assess in many elderly because of arthritic effects on the hand and wrist and because it is not able to reflect loss of function of the lower body.

Standardized physical performance measures complement the measures of muscle mass for the assessment of sarcopenia. Physical performance measures are correlated with body composition and skeletal muscle parameters and predict relevant health-related outcomes, such as mortality, morbidity, institutionalization, and disability.[5,13] The short physical performance battery (SPPB), gait speed at usual pace over a short distance, the long corridor walking test (400-m walk test), and the 6-minute walk test are among the most widely used and validated measures.[5,17–20] Another useful physical performance measure is the stair climb test.[19] Among this wide range of physical performance tests, SPPB and gait speed have recently been recommended for clinical trials in frail older adults.[20] Levels of clinically meaningful change have been established for the SPPB (1 point) and gait speed (0.10 m/s on a 4-m walking test).[21,22] In addition, SPPB and gait speed have demonstrated excellent reliability, predictive validity for a large number of adverse outcomes, including mortality, nursing home admission, hospitalization, falls, and new onset of disability, and sensitivity to clinically important change.[5,20]

BIOLOGICAL MARKERS IN TRIALS

Adipose tissue produces several adipokines (such as leptin) and proinflammatory cytokines (such as tumor necrosis factor α and interleukins 1 and 6), all of which are associated with aging, obesity, and sarcopenia. Several studies have shown independent associations of these factors with lower muscle strength, lower physical performance, and higher risk of disability in older persons.[13] Assessment of antioxidants, such as intake of carotenoids and vitamin C and plasma levels of α- and γ-tocopherols, is inversely associated with measures of sarcopenia. Several other biomarkers have shown significant associations with measures of sarcopenia. Anemia is associated with lower muscle strength and physical performance in older persons, and low serum albumin levels are associated with poor grip strength in older men and women.[13] Vitamin D plays an important role in the skeletal muscle metabolism, and persons with low serum 25-hydroxyvitamin D levels have poor muscle mass measured with DXA and diminished lower grip strength.[23] Therefore, several studies have shown that adipokines, proinflammatory cytokines, markers of oxidative damage, and a broad range of other biomarkers have strong and independent associations with several measures of sarcopenia. However, such markers are also associated with a wide range of other diseases and conditions. Depending on the overall goal of the trial, biomarkers should be included. The use of blood sampling and dosing biomarkers in large preventive trials depends on specific end points and costs.[10] In the case of smaller sample sizes in intervention trials, blood sampling is possible and probably needed to eliminate possible confounders that could diminish the expected effect of an intervention.

END POINTS FOR TRIALS IN SARCOPENIA

Primary outcomes for clinical trials of interventions on sarcopenia should be highly responsive to treatment effects and clinically relevant. Functional abilities are the most clinically relevant factors affected by sarcopenia, and the primary end point of all sarcopenia trials should include the assessment of physical performances.[22] Among performance-based measures of function, the best-studied measures are those that assess the function and mobility of lower extremity, which contains the largest muscles of the body. Such measures have demonstrated predictive validity for numerous critical health factors such as survival, health care use, future functional decline, and quality of life. Performance measures of mobility have also repeatedly been shown to be sensitive to changes in strength.[22] After identifying a valid and reliable assessment tool as a primary end point, a clinically meaningful change detected by the tool becomes an issue and needs to be identified. Without this identified meaningful change, the intervention is considered clinically relevant even if statistically significant.[10] As stated earlier, SPPB and gait speed (over a short distance at usual pace) are recommended as the primary end points in clinical trials.[20] However, another challenge with function-related end points is that disability fluctuates and is variable among older adults, especially among those related to transient acute illness and exacerbations of chronic illness. Investigators should cope with eventual fluctuations of end points, and the best analytic strategies should be proposed to minimize the effect of fluctuation. Although time-to-event designs with survival analyses are currently being used, analyses by linear mixed effects models have been proposed for data that are repeatedly assessed in longitudinal cohorts and might fluctuate over time.[24]

In trials involving sarcopenia, in order to determine if the treatment worked the way it was expected to, strength and muscle mass need to be assessed as secondary end points. Clearly, all the issues that affect strength and mass measurements including validity, feasibility, and reproducibility come into play if they are to be considered as secondary end points and of particular interest in specific research areas and intervention trials.[22] Investigators need to be selective in the possible secondary end points to include confounders but to avoid participant burden in old-aged population.[10] Some end points are not applicable to all participants. Incapacity to perform an end point assessment (for example, in the case of disabled older adults unable to perform a physical performance assessment) automatically transforms it into an exclusion criterion, and the older adults who cannot perform the end points of the trial cannot be enrolled. In these cases, the development of new scales or end points for special subpopulations should be encouraged or the secondary end point should not be included in the trial.

Special attention also needs to be taken regarding cognition because trials involving physical activity, physical performance, and strength could affect progression of cognitive decline and adherence to the protocol, compliance with the interventions, and programmed follow-up could be influenced by cognitive status.[25,26] In a sarcopenia trial, a general recommendation could be to assess cognition, at baseline and during follow-up, and to evaluate direct and indirect drug effects on cognitive decline over time.

Fat mass contributes significantly to functional impairment in elderly people independent of muscle mass, and sarcopenic obesity was associated with an increased mobility disability compared with sarcopenia without obesity.[27] It is possible that the combination of high fat mass and low muscle mass is detrimental and highly predictive of functional decline. Changes over time in the fat mass could predict increases or decreases in future sarcopenia-related impairments, and intervention could be effective by changing fat mass with no initial effects on muscle mass. Until the exact physiopathologic pathways are known, it is recommended to measure and take into account fat mass in analytic strategies as a confounder. Also, intramuscular adipose infiltration is related to increasing age and increasing fat mass among different racial groups, and it is associated with metabolic abnormalities, poor strength, and performance measurers, as well as incident mobility disability and higher concentrations of inflammatory markers.[28,29] Reduction of adipose infiltration by intervention could increase performance without a significant change in muscular mass. In cases in which the expected drug effect is to reduce adipose infiltration, MRI or CT scans could be proposed as a secondary end point and as a biomarker of drug efficacy.

DESIGN OF INTERVENTIONS IN PHASE 3 TRIALS

To verify the efficacy of interventions, it is important to maximize potential benefit and minimize possible toxicity. For complex syndromes, such as sarcopenia in older populations, multidomain intervention trials are being proposed in which several combined intervention approaches in one group are compared with alternative combined interventions or controls in another group. The main issue to be resolved in such trials is the interpretation of the results because it is difficult to assess which individual intervention did or did not work. Interventions such as drugs, nutrition, programs of physical exercising, and social interventions depend on the type of trial and its feasibility. In order for evidence in a clinical trial to determine relevant difference from an intervention, usual clinical care (present in both intervention and control groups) needs to be characterized and standardized without contaminating the control group. Interventions also need to be standardized and be strong enough to be sufficiently relevant because the usual care in the control group is enhanced due to participation in a clinical trial.[30] Physical activity remains an issue because it is sometimes considered usual care and sometimes an intervention depending on the trial. So whether exercise is considered usual care and should be promoted in both control and intervention groups is an unresolved issue when enrolling sedentary older participants in a trial. Therefore, assessment of self-reported physical activity by a structured questionnaire should be systematically required in all trials even if inconsistencies are associated with the assessment.

DESIGNING A PHASE 3 PREVENTIVE TRIAL ON SARCOPENIA

Many aspects of the design of a preventive trial on sarcopenia have been discussed herein. Table 3 shows the main characteristics of such trials. Briefly, presarcopenic (solely based on low muscle mass) adults older than 70 years, DXA (body composition assessment), hand grip (strength), gait speed and SPPB (physical performance), delayed sarcopenia onset (as primary end points: muscle mass, strength, or physical performance), and inclusion of all possible confounders (as secondary end points), by providing few exclusion criteria, are the basis for a preventive trial. The trial must have a randomized control design, with the control group defined as "best standard of usual clinical care."[10] Multidomain interventions (interventions in different areas at the same time) for the prevention of sarcopenia should be used based on the existence of multiple physiopathologic pathways of sarcopenia onset and progression in older adults.[11,22] Finally, follow-up should be standardized based on the overall goal. A broad recommendation of a 6-month follow-up can be settled, with a total duration of the trial of 1 to 3 years (depending on primary end point, population characteristics, and feasibility), taking into account annual rate of decline in physical performance, muscle mass, and strength.

DESIGNING A PHASE 3 INTERVENTION TRIAL ON SARCOPENIA

Many aspects of the design of an intervention trial on sarcopenia have been discussed previously. Table 3 shows the main characteristics of such trials. Briefly, sarcopenic (low muscle mass and low physical performance or strength) adults older than 70 years, DXA, MRI or CT (for body composition assessment), complex strength and physical performance measures, treatment of sarcopenia (primary end point being physical performance), strength and muscle mass (as secondary end points), and the inclusion of the fewest possible confounders (as secondary end points) by increasing exclusion criteria are the basis of an intervention trial. The homogenization

Table 3
Design of phase 3 trials in sarcopenia

	Preventive Trial on Sarcopenia	Intervention Trial on Sarcopenia
Overall Goal	Delay the onset of sarcopenia	Treat sarcopenia
Sarcopenia Definition	Presarcopenia: low muscle mass with normal strength and physical performance	Sarcopenia: low muscle mass with decreased strength or physical performance Severe sarcopenia: low muscle mass with decreased strength and physical performance
Muscle Mass Assessment	DXA	DXA, MRI, or CT
Strength Assessment	Hand grip	Hand grip, complex isokinetic strength measures of power and torque
Physical Performance Assessment	Gait speed, SPPB	Gait speed, SPPB, LCWT, 6-minute walking test, stair climb test
Screening Population	Adults older than 70 years Autonomous adults Community-dwelling adults Normal strength and physical performance	Adults older than 70 years Autonomous or disabled adults Community-dwelling adults or specific communities Acute conditions such as falls, hospitalization, or selective surgery Impairments in strength and physical performance
Target Population	Broad sarcopenia definition No restrictive inclusion/exclusion criteria Heterogeneous population (solely based on muscle mass measurements) Large population Generalization to whole aging population if intervention effective	Restrictive sarcopenia definition Restrictive inclusion/exclusion criteria Homogeneous population Smaller population than a preventive trial Generalization to whole aging population will be an issue
Possible Confounders	Inactivity/physical activity Nutrition Previous disability Demography (gender, age, ethnicity) Chronic conditions (diseases and drugs) Biological markers (adipokines, inflammatory markers, vitamin D, etc)	
Primary End Points	Delay the onset of decline or increase physical performance and strength Stop decline or increase muscle mass	Increase physical performance

Secondary End Points	• Limit secondary outcomes to avoid overburden
	  ○ Onset of permanent disabilities (ADL)
	  ○ Onset of cognitive decline
	  ○ Mortality
	  ○ Institutionalization
	  ○ Hospitalization
	• Changes in cognition
	• Changes in fat mass
	• Evolution of biomarkers over time (if available)
	• Falls
	• Quality of life
		Few secondary outcomes
		Increase muscle mass
		Increase strength
		Evolution of biomarkers over time
		Changes in cognition
		Changes in fat infiltration
		Changes in fat mass

(continued on next page)

Table 3 (continued)	Preventive Trial on Sarcopenia	Intervention Trial on Sarcopenia
Trial design	Randomized controlled trial Control group: best standard of care	Randomized controlled trial Control group: best standard of care
Intervention	Multidomain intervention Single-drug intervention Standardized program of physical activity	Single-drug intervention Standardized program of physical activity
Duration	1–3 y	12–18 mo

Abbreviation: ADL, activities of daily living.

of the enrolled population powers the study, traducing a sample size reduction with an increasing chance of proving effectiveness of the intervention.

Once more, the trial must be a randomized controlled one, with the control group defined as the best standard of usual clinical care. The intervention should generally be a single intervention (mainly drug intervention). Although contamination of the control group is less probable, exercising becomes an issue if considered as usual care, and investigators will need to standardize physical activity during trial design. Specific subgroups might participate in the trial, and dependency needs to be accounted for.[10]

Trial duration and follow-up depend on treatment properties, but should generally be conducted over a 12- to 18-month period.

HEALTH CARE COSTS OF SARCOPENIA

The sarcopenia-related economic burden is because of the links of low muscle mass with poor physical functioning, disability onset, and mortality.[31–33] Loss in physical function increases even more the risk of physical disability, along with increased nursing home admission and mortality.[2,34] Therefore, sarcopenia is responsible for approximately $18 billion annual direct health care costs in the United States.[35] To put this in perspective, it has been estimated that the yearly economic cost of osteoporotic fractures in the United States is $16.3 billion.[36] Considering that the total number of older adults is expected to double over the next 25 years, the absolute costs associated with sarcopenia are expected to increase sharply.[9] Conducting phase 3 clinical trials, even if challenging, could eventually generate new strategies to prevent or treat sarcopenia and its associated health consequences. These strategies could ultimately reduce the health care costs along with an increase in quality of life of the elderly.

SUMMARY

- The design of sarcopenia trials is challenging but worthwhile because progression of the disabling process of older adults can be intervened upon.
- Current research on the plausible mechanistic pathways leading to sarcopenia and the functional consequences of sarcopenia are hampered by a lack of a consensus definition and a standardized assessment methodology.
- Taking into account the prevalence of sarcopenia in community-dwelling older adults, the target population could be established at an age of 70 years or more.
- Physical performance measures should be considered as the main end points.
- Physical exercising, whether considered as usual care or intervention, remains an issue.

- The most commonly used, low cost, and accessible method to assess skeletal muscle mass is DXA.

REFERENCES

1. Rosenberg IH. Summary comments. Am J Clin Nutr 1989;50:1231–3.
2. Abellan van Kan G. Epidemiology and consequences of sarcopenia. J Nutr Health Aging 2009;13(8):708–12.
3. Pahor M, Cesari M. Designing phase IIB trials in sarcopenia. The best target population. J Nutr Health Aging 2011. DOI: 10.1007/s12603-011-0058-9.
4. Cruz-Jentoft A, Baeyens JP, Bauer J, et al. Sarcopenia: European consensus on definition and diagnosis: report of the European working group on sarcopenia in older people. Age Ageing 2010;39:412–23.
5. Abellan van Kan G, Rolland Y, Andrieu S, et al. Gait speed at usual pace as a predictor of adverse outcomes in community-dwelling older people an International Academy on Nutrition and Aging (IANA) task force. J Nutr Health Aging 2009;13(10):881–9.
6. Thomas DR. Sarcopenia. Clin Geriatr Med 2010;26(2):331–46.
7. Clark BC, Manini TM. Sarcopenia =/= dynapenia. J Gerontol A Biol Sci Med Sci 2008;63(8):829–34.
8. Visser M. Towards a definition of sarcopenia. Results from epidemiological studies. J Nutr Health Aging 2009;13(8):713–6.
9. Clark BC, Manini TM. Functional consequences of sarcopenia and dynapenia in the elderly. Curr Opin Clin Nutr Metab Care 2010;13:271–6.
10. Abellan van Kan G, André E, Bischoff-Ferrari HA, et al. Carla task force on sarcopenia: propositions for clinical trials. J Nutr Health Aging 2009;13(8):700–7.
11. Studenski S. Target populations for clinical trials. J Nutr Health Aging 2009;13(8): 729–32.
12. Morley JE. Sarcopenia: diagnosis and treatment. J Nutr Health Aging 2008;12(7): 452–6.
13. Pahor M, Manini T, Cesari M. Sarcopenia: clinical evaluation, biological markers and other evaluation tools. J Nutr Health Aging 2009;13(8):724–8.
14. Cesari M, Leeuwenburgh C, Lauretani F, et al. Frailty syndrome and skeletal muscle: results from the Invecchiare in Chianti study. Am J Clin Nutr 2006; 83(5):1142–8.
15. Newman AB, Kupelian V, Visser M, et al. Strength, but not muscle mass, is associated with mortality in the health, aging and body composition study cohort. J Gerontol A Biol Sci Med Sci 2006;61(1):72–7.
16. Lauretani F, Russo C, Bandinelli S, et al. Age-associated change in skeletal muscles and their effect on mobility: an operational definition of sarcopenia. J Appl Physiol 2003;95:1851–60.
17. Guralnik JM, Ferrucci L, Simonsick EM, et al. Lower-extremity function in persons over the age of 70 years as a predictor of subsequent disability. N Engl J Med 1995;332(9):556–61.
18. Newman AB, Simonsick EM, Naydeck EM, et al. Association of long-distance corridor walk performance with mortality, cardiovascular disease, mobility limitation, and disability. JAMA 2006;295(17):2018–26.
19. Ettinger WH, Burns R, Messier SP, et al. The Fitness Arthritis and Seniors Trial (FAST): a randomized trial comparing aerobic exercise and resistance exercise to a health education program on physical disability in older people with knee osteoarthritis. JAMA 1997;277:25–31.

20. Working Group on Functional Outcome Measures for Clinical Trials. Functional outcomes for clinical trials in frail older persons. Time to be moving. J Gerontol A Biol Sci Med Sci 2008;63(2):160–4.

21. Perera S, Mody SH, Woodman RC, et al. Meaningful change and responsiveness in common physical performance measures in older adults. J Am Geriatr Soc 2006;54:743–9.

22. Studenski S. What are the outcomes of treatment among patents with sarcopenia? J Nutr Health Aging 2009;13(8):733–6.

23. Visser M, Deeg DJ, Lips P. Low vitamin D and high parathyroid hormone levels as determinants of loss of muscle strength and muscle mass (sarcopenia): the longitudinal aging study Amsterdam. J Clin Endocrinol Metab 2003;88(12):5766–72.

24. Carrière I, Bouyer J. Choosing marginal or random-effects models for longitudinal binary responses: application to self-reported disability among older persons. BMC Med Res Methodol 2002;2:15.

25. Williamson JD, Espeland M, Kritchevsky SB, et al. Changes in cognitive function in a randomized trial of physical activity: results of the lifestyle interventions and independence for elders pilot study. J Gerontol A Biol Sci Med Sci 2009;64(6):688–94.

26. Rolland Y, Abellan van Kan G, Vellas B. Healthy brain aging: role of exercise and physical activity. Clin Geriatr Med 2010;26(1):75–87.

27. Rolland Y, Lauwers-Cances V, Cristini C, et al. Difficulties with physical function associated with obesity, sarcopenia, and sarcopenic-obesity in community-dwelling elderly women: the EPIDOS (EPIDemiologie de l'OSteoporose) study. Am J Clin Nutr 2009;89:1895–900.

28. Zoico E, Rossi A, Di Francesco V, et al. Adipose tissue infiltration in skeletal muscle of healthy elderly men: relationships with body composition, insulin resistance, and inflammation at the systemic and tissue level. J Gerontol A Biol Sci Med Sci 2010;65A(3):295–9.

29. Beasley LE, Koster A, Newman AB, et al. Inflammation and race and gender differences in computerized tomography-measured adipose depots. Obesity (Silver Spring) 2009;17:1062–9.

30. Nourhashemi F, Andrieu S, Gillette-Guyonnet S, et al. Effectiveness of a specific care plan in patients with Alzheimer's disease: cluster randomised trial (PLASA study). BMJ 2010;340:c2466.

31. Reid KF, Naumova EN, Carabello RJ, et al. Lower extremity muscle mass predicts functional performance in mobility-limited elders. J Nutr Health Aging 2008;12: 493–8.

32. Janssen I, Baumgartner RN, Ross R, et al. Skeletal muscle cutpoints associated with elevated physical disability risk in older men and women. Am J Epidemiol 2004;159:413–21.

33. Kimyagarov S, Klid R, Levenkrohn S, et al. Body mass index, body composition and mortality of nursing home elderly residents. Arch Gerontol Geriatr 2010;51(2): 227–30.

34. Guralnik JM, Ferrucci L, Pieper CF, et al. Lower extremity function and subsequent disability: consistency across studies, predictive models, and value of gait speed alone compared with the short physical performance battery. J Gerontol A Biol Sci Med Sci 2000;55(4):221–31.

35. Janssen I, Shepard DS, Katzmarzyk PT, et al. The healthcare cost of sarcopenia in the United States. J Am Geriatr Soc 2004;52:80–5.

36. Ray NF, Chan JK, Thamer M, et al. Medical expenditures for the treatment of osteoporotic fractures in the United States in 1995. Report from the National Osteoporosis Foundation. J Bone Miner Res 1997;12:24–35.

Index

Clin Geriatr Med 27 (2011) 483–489
Doi:10.1016/S0749-0690(11)00059-0
0749-0690/11/$ – see front matter © 2011 Elsevier Inc. All rights reserved.

geriatric.theclinics.com

Moving?

Make sure your subscription moves with you!

To notify us of your new address, find your **Clinics Account Number** (located on your mailing label above your name), and contact customer service at:

Email: journalscustomerservice-usa@elsevier.com

800-654-2452 (subscribers in the U.S. & Canada)
314-447-8871 (subscribers outside of the U.S. & Canada)

Fax number: 314-447-8029

Elsevier Health Sciences Division
Subscription Customer Service
3251 Riverport Lane
Maryland Heights, MO 63043

*To ensure uninterrupted delivery of your subscription,
please notify us at least 4 weeks in advance of move.

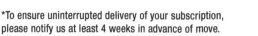
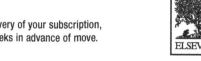

ELSEVIER

Printed in the United States
By Bookmasters